YES
YOU
CAN

A HELPBOOK FOR THE
PHYSICALLY DISABLED

YES
YOU
CAN

Helynn Hoffa and Gary Morgan

PHAROS BOOKS
A SCRIPPS HOWARD COMPANY
NEW YORK

Portions of this book have previously appeared, some in somewhat different form, in *Accent on Living* magazine, *Together* magazine, the Raleigh (N.C.) *Spectator* magazine, and *Mainstream* magazine, have been included on CompuServe's Handicapped Users' Database and in CompuServe's Disabilities Forum, and are included here by permission of the authors and those organizations.

First published in 1990.

Library of Congress Cataloging-in-Publication Data:
Hoffa, Helynn.
    Yes you can : a helpbook for the physically disabled / Helynn
Hoffa and Gary Morgan.
        p.   cm.
    Includes index.
    ISBN 0-88687-480-7
    1. Physically handicapped—United States—Life skills guides.
I. Morgan, Gary.   II. Title.
    HV3023.A3H64   1990
    362.4—dc20   90-43239
                                                       CIP

Printed in the United States of America.

Jacket and interior design by Bea Jackson

Pharos Books
A Scripps Howard Company
200 Park Avenue
New York, New York 10166

10 9 8 7 6 5 4 3 2 1

This book is dedicated to the memory of Gini Laurie, whose practical dedication to the disabled has touched all our lives, whether we knew her or not.

◆ ACKNOWLEDGMENTS ◆

No project of this sort could ever be attempted without the help and encouragement of a great many people. We are deeply indebted and grateful for the contribution of everyone mentioned in this book and to many others who gave of their time, effort, and support.

Our thanks to Cyndi Jones of *Mainstream* magazine, to Betty Garee of *Accent on Living* magazine, to Joan Headley of the International Polio Network, and especially to freelance writer Sharon Whitley, who served as Helynn's interviewer and research assistant. Thanks, too, to Steve Hier for converting Apple-format data files to IBM for us.

We are extremely grateful to Christine Sackey, who helped organize and assemble the resource guide at the end of this book. Special thanks to Georgia Griffith, deaf and blind operator of CompuServe's Handicapped Users' Database, who helped readily with any question or problem and usually found an answer the same day. In addition, we gratefully acknowledge the help and cooperation of CompuServe Information Service and its people, especially Kitty Munger Thomas, Pat Phelps, and Dave Manning, who went out of their way to make sure information was complete and current.

Finally, we thank our agent, Mark Frisk of the Howard Buck Agency, for his tireless faith in this project, and our editor, Shari Jee, who kept our ideas focused.

Without the help and faith of each and every one of you this book would not have been possible. Thank you!

HELYNN HOFFA
GARY MORGAN

CONTENTS

I was sitting on the steps by the pool at Warm Springs, Georgia, one morning when Franklin D. Roosevelt came swimming over. We chitchatted for a few minutes—about my progress, about the Depression, and about the value of this polio treatment center he had built for the thousands like us. Then he stopped and looked at me for a minute.

"What do you want to be when you grow up?" he asked finally.

I shrugged and told him I wasn't sure I could "be" anything, but that if I had a choice, I'd like to be an archeologist.

"Just remember this," he said softly. "If I can be in a wheelchair and be president of the greatest country in the world, you can do or be whatever you want to be."

That encounter with FDR when I was twelve has guided me ever since. Here was a person, I thought, who had to deal with the same things I had to deal with. And he had to run the United States, too.

I never became an archeologist; it was an unrealistic choice. First, it was unrealistic for me to think I could go to dusty deserts or fetid jungles to dig up ancient things, however adventurous and exciting that might sound. Two, I had no practical guidelines to follow. It was, however, much better than no choice at all. A life with no goal, no objective, is a rudderless life.

I continued going to public school in my wheelchair and worked hard to learn as much as I could and to keep my grades up. I was rarely in the classroom more than two and a half days a week, if that often, because of my health. With the teachers' cooperation (all were helpful), I handed in my homework and took every test. I was smart enough to realize that an education was essential to gain whatever opportunities I might have in life.

My education was often interrupted by trips to doctors in both the United States and Canada and by prolonged stays in children's orthopedic hospitals. My determination to walk again was relentless. It drove me like an obsession, but to no avail. My physical condition did not improve; instead, I tired from overexertion. I was unwilling to face either adolescence or adulthood in a wheelchair. But face it I did.

Growing up in a small town (Sunbury, Pennsylvania, had a stable population of 16,000) had many advantages, most of them social. Children and adults alike accepted me, and I became a part of the social scene. Although it often happens to disabled children and adults, I was never the "odd man out." But there was no "higher education," nothing beyond high school. Even worse, no one knew anything about archeology!

The State of Pennsylvania, in an experiment in rehabilitation, gave me an IQ test, determined that I ranked just above the genius level, and offered to pay all my expenses in the school of journalism at the University of Pennsylvania in Philadelphia. I was ecstatic. Then the blow fell. The offer hinged on the publisher of our local paper promising to hire me for one year. He said no! I had lost my chance at college and vowed to leave Sunbury.

For the first time in my life I was bitter. The twin blows of losing my chance for a college education and the realization that I would never walk were difficult to cope with at nineteen. Or any age, for that matter.

But the words of FDR came back to me over and over again: "You can be whatever you want to be." I clung to them for dear life. It was a dark time for me.

Education became of paramount importance. And books are always available, of course. I took my first correspondence course through the University of Chicago. I studied Egyptology. The school sent me a list of books, and I dove into the waters of self-education. Some years later I was a student at the University of California, Berkeley, and at Southwestern Community College (a junior college I helped bring into existence through my work in politics).

I learned that if one course of action isn't possible, I could always change tactics. But I couldn't afford to quit. When you quit, you're slamming a door shut; when you change tactics (or direction), you're opening another one. The object is to open as many doors as possible, especially if you're disabled. Once a door has been closed, it isn't easy to reopen.

My parents went into civil service and we moved to Pearl Harbor, Hawaii. I continued my activities in the Polio Foundation's March of Dimes, and I also joined the Cruising Club of Hawaii. The next year, I spearheaded the March of Dimes and the yacht club elected me historian. Through the ensuing publicity, I got a job as a sports reporter on the Honolulu *Star-Bulletin*. I kept the job because I had "paid my dues" by reading, writing, and studying. Doors kept opening, and I became editor of *Hawaiian Sportsman* magazine, took over a Sunday-night radio program about sport fishing and yachting news, wrote a children's book and a book of poetry and dozens of magazine articles on a wide range of subjects—from Hawaiian history to "How to Plan a Nautical Luncheon."

After moving to California I turned my attention back to my original goal and enrolled at UC Berkeley with an anthropology major and minors in political science and English literature. I did the required laboratory work (in biology, geography, and the other sciences) at Southwestern Community College. It kept me busy, but I still needed to earn money. So I became bookkeeper for my church, taught children's art classes Saturday mornings and Oriental art classes to adults on weekdays. Fortunately, I had taken classes at the Honolulu Academy of Fine Arts. In the years since, I've been able to do many things—from being a sports writer to ceramicist to print shop operator. Most important, I've been able to make my way in the world. But I've had to struggle.

This book is based on my struggles; it is written to save other people the years I wasted while I floundered around not knowing how to work toward a goal. I desperately needed an easy-to-follow practical book of advice and some blueprints to help me succeed.

I hope this book will provide those blueprints. It is designed to help, in practical terms, everyone who reads it. It is about what aid is available today, both public and private. It is also about planning to succeed. Everyone can succeed at something. Every life can be productive, satisfying, and worth living. All that's needed is desire, enthusiasm, and knowledge. You can provide the desire and enthusiasm; I'll help with the knowledge.

Just remember: you can be whatever you want to be.

HELYNN HOFFA
La Jolla, Calif.
April 1990

So the Unthinkable Has Happened to You

A physical handicap is hardly something we plan on in advance; it happens whether we are ready for it or not. The unexpected is always unsettling, of course, because we are never truly prepared to deal with it. In the best of circumstances, it can leave us uncertain, bewildered, disconnected, and confused. Up to this time, you've been busy learning the rules of the game of life. Now, suddenly, all the rules have changed abruptly. They changed when a doctor said, "You have muscular dystrophy" or "The dive broke your neck" or "The car wreck injured your spinal column" or "We had to remove both legs."

You don't hear him the first time. The reality of his words is too awful to assimilate, so your ears close to the sound of his voice. Or your mind shuts down. Or, if the words get through, you don't believe them. After all, doctors have been wrong before—plenty wrong. They don't have an exclusive on correct diagnoses. Everyone knows that. And you're sure that he *is* wrong this time.

You tell yourself, "This isn't happening to me." You console yourself with "I'll be out of here in a couple of days. Right as rain. Good as new." Over and over again, you think "This is just some minor temporary glitch." Tomorrow you'll be back to normal.

Friends drop by during visiting hours, with funny looks on their faces. They bring flowers, candy (for the nurses, since they usually wind up eating it anyway), books, and strained conversation.

A bookkeeper stops in. He wants to know how you plan to pay the shockingly high bill.

A social worker wants to know what arrangements are being made to care for you at home.

A physiotherapist begins teaching you exercises and says, "These must be done every day so your muscles don't atrophy."

All day it goes on—breakfast brought in on a tray, the nurse helping you wash, the lab technician drawing enough blood to float a small ship. Later, an orderly manhandles you onto a gurney, more X-rays are taken, doctors—ones you haven't seen before—pop in eager to have a look. Then comes an inedible lunch and more of the morning routine in the afternoon. Only the sleeping pill at night turns off the daily round of indignities.

You long for privacy. You cling to the memories of it. A condition you probably never thought about before becomes the most important thing in your life and commands your attention during virtually all of your waking hours. Resentment toward the people around you—not only the hospital staff but your friends and relatives as well—begins to build up. They are all crowding you, stripping you of every minute, intruding on your solitude.

"As soon as I get out of this madhouse, I'm going backpacking in the Adirondacks—alone!" This you vow as the pill finally takes effect and you slip, mercifully, into sleep.

Getting help—when it matters

A person becomes physically disabled in one of three ways: being born with a defect, falling victim to a crippling disease like muscular dystrophy, or suffering an accident. Helynn has found that the psychological problems generally are the same, varying more according to the personalities of the individuals than the physical differences generated by the handicap. A strong, innovative person appears, on the surface at least, to make the necessary adjustments with more ease and efficiency than the one who finds problem-solving both difficult and tiresome, just as the pre-teen with the natural exuberance of the young seems to cope better than the adult.

The teen years and the early twenties are probably the most difficult ages for dealing with physical disabilities. These are usually the years of strenuous physical activity, a time to test the boundaries of personal achievement and the development of body, mind, and ego—all difficult enough to cope with in the best of circumstances. Add a physical handicap or life-threatening disease and a volatile situation can develop quickly. Counseling provided by social workers, psychologists, and psychiatrists can help salvage the most battered ego, and this book will suggest ways of approaching counseling to ensure that it yields the greatest advantage.

In every case, the sooner professional help is secured, the better. The road ahead is largely uncharted for the disabled person—and signposts are rare. Without some direction, too many mistakes can be made too easily. Life requires direction for a person to mature, to know the satisfaction of accomplishment; without goals, living loses its zest and becomes a monotonous counting of the days on the calendar. Yesterday you knew where you were going to school, what career you would pursue, how you would live. Today all that is gone. What lies ahead is uncertain. But what's inside you *is* certain. You can look deep inside yourself and dredge up the courage to change your life, to put order into what is suddenly chaos. We hope the suggestions here will help restore some order, too.

While self-assurance and self-confidence may come from somewhere deep inside you, it cannot possibly hurt to motivate, encourage, and otherwise aid and abet the growth of these badly needed attributes. Everyone with a handicap can benefit from psychological help (even though the natural tendency is to resist it) whether the physical obstacles stem from birth defects, disease, or accident. The social and economic situations caused by these tragedies are the same for everyone, no matter what an individual's physical condition and no matter when and how it changes. A trained professional can help with the adjustment.

What the doctor ordered

Proper medical aid is equally important. Following the doctor's orders and the physical therapist's instructions is imperative. Later this book suggests important things to bear in mind when dealing with this vital area. For now, though, remember: If for any reason you aren't comfortable with your doctor or physical therapist (or your psychologist, or anyone else, for that matter), change to someone else. Just don't give up on the process, even though it might seem tedious and unproductive at times. These people—the doctors, therapists, nurses, psychologists—have become vital not only to your existence, but also to the quality of that existence. It will be the only existence you get, so make the most of it. To do anything else would be foolhardy.

Don't try to be needlessly brave or enduring, either. If your medicine makes you sick, upsets your stomach, or causes head-ache or dizziness, talk to your physician. Do it right away. Don't wait days or weeks to do something about it and, above all, don't just stop taking the medication. Call the doctor's office and leave a message. The doctor will call you back later in the day. Chances are he or she can adjust your dosage on the phone or switch your medication with a simple call to the pharmacist. If the exercises tire your muscles or cause pain, tell your rehabilitation technician or physical therapist. He or she can modify the routine. If your psychotherapist upsets you or doesn't seem to make sense, change to another. On the other hand, if you reach a point where the sessions don't seem to help, stick it out a bit longer. Chances are you're over the hump and about to be discharged from care.

Your life is still up to you

All these things are important to your preparation for a new kind of life—important not just to your existence but for a happy, rewarding, and successful life, the kind of life we all strive for and expect to attain. After all that's happened, can you still have that? Yes. It can still be yours—if you're as willing to work for it now as you were before the catastrophe. That's the key. What you make of your life has always been up to you. It still is. That hasn't changed.

The length of time it takes to adjust to the major changes ordained by the irrevocable physical catastrophe depends on the determination of the individual. The sooner you decide to take charge of your life, the better for you. And the better for your family and friends. It may not have occurred to you during those dark times you spent in the pit of despondency, but those who love and care for you are enmeshed in this disaster, too. They don't know how to handle it either, and they will display a natural tendency to take their cue from you. In other words, they will react to your condition in much the same way you do.

At first, usually depending on the severity of your handicap, your family and close friends will react in one of two ways: They will either become oversolicitous or will flee the scene. Both reactions can drive you to the brink of distraction. If for no other reason than your own peace of mind, you have to take the initiative and put them at ease. This book will offer some ways to do just that. As a rule, however, you should bear in mind that your friends aren't going to consult your battery of medical, physical, and mental advisers. All they know is what you say and how you behave. Give them a break—they're your closest allies.

While you are struggling to sort all this out, you have to begin thinking about your future at some point. You do have one, you know, and no one but you can decide what it is going to include. Life is a process of going from here to there. There are maps, certainly, but there are no guarantees. The society we are born into provides a variety of guidelines: family, church, school, and government. If we are physically normal, of average intelligence, and willing to learn, we do well; but on occasion an unexpected roadblock looms unavoidably on the path we've planned. Then drastic changes have to be worked out quickly and put into action.

Let your intuition be your guide

In life, as in mathematics, you must first postulate and identify the problems created by your physical handicap, then you can propose rules for overcoming them. Until the problem has been defined, finding a solution is impossible. While problem solving demands analysis, logic, and a dispassionate view of reality, it also requires imagination. Don't overlook intuition, and don't ever sell your dreams short. Without those dreams, whatever you achieve will contain a hollow core.

Problem solving needn't be a difficult or obscure exercise. We'll help guide you through the process by developing lists and setting goals. Whether you are young and just now trying to choose a profession or older and forced to make a midcareer goal change, the procedures are basically the same and should be made using all the physical, mental, and philosophical tools available. The goal must be realistic and the steps toward its fulfillment must be possible. In the Anglican church there is a saying: "To become a religious [a priest, monk, nun, or the like] three things are required: The call, the means, the place."

The same can be said of goals in the secular scene. You must have a genuine desire to accomplish something in your life, and you must have a definite goal. The sorrow is not in failing to reach the goal; it lies in not trying. Life without direction is meaningless, and in its meaninglessness it is without satisfaction. Trust in your dreams and ambitions, but curb your impossible daydreams. Vast differences separate dreams and daydreams: The first will aid you, the second will betray you. It isn't difficult to distinguish between them. The spotlight of common-sense reality will banish the impossible daydreams and illuminate the dreams.

Education: Skills for living

After the medical and emotional problems are faced and the programs to deal with them established, it is time to consider education. Without a skill or a profession, life becomes a daily round of such minor indulgences as overeating, drinking, and watching endless hours of television. The gratification gleaned from these nonactivities lessens as the months and years go on. Giving up the effort it takes to improve your circumstances is easy, but if you do you'll live to regret it. Sloth is deceptive, especially in your situation.

Education actually begins when we are born and doesn't end until we die: It is an ongoing set of experiences. Some experiences we have no say in or control over; we just have to meet them head-on the best way we know how. We generally call them elements of "the school of hard knocks." The drifters stay in this school. "It is easier," they say. "And, besides, why make decisions or plans? They aren't going to work out the way I want them to anyway."

Failure. It's inevitable. And with it comes self-pity. "What the hell can I do?" you think when it happens. "The cards are stacked against me. I can't get out of bed. I can't get out of a wheelchair. I have multiple sclerosis (or a severed spinal column or polio or whatever). So I'm taking medication, doing exercises, seeing a psychiatrist, praying. What more is there?"

Well, there is education. A whetstone upon which to hone your mind. The theme of a United Negro College Fund campaign is "A mind is a terrible thing to waste." This applies to everyone, equally, in every country, no matter what the social or economic situation. The more education a person has, the easier it is to cope with life's problems and the greater the chance for fulfillment. Education opens doors, makes options available, and draws roadmaps; it also delights, confounds, and illuminates; it puzzles, wearies, and challenges. But it never bores.

Education comes in a variety of packages, large and small, depending on what you want from it. Other than that which is thrust on us willy-nilly by the circumstances of life and the state's requirements of a certain basic amount of schooling, we are free to choose the sort of education we want. Give yourself an advantage: Choose a college education. But beware. A college catalog presents the would-be student with such a dazzling array of subjects that it is impossible to choose without an agenda.

Ellen J. has been a college student for some time, but she lacks an agenda. She said in an interview, "I've been going to community colleges for five years and still don't have an associate degree in anything."

"Why not?" Helynn asked. "Do you get failing grades or do you drop classes?"

"Neither," she said hesitantly. She gave a self-conscious sigh. "The courses all look so interesting that it's difficult to decide what to take. So I choose whatever strikes my fancy without paying attention to the requirements for my major."

"You're what is known as a professional sophomore," Helynn told her.

"I know. But one of these semesters I'll transfer to a university and get a B.A."

She hasn't done it yet, and she won't until she recognizes that side trips to "interesting" courses are short vacations from the more serious job of reaching a goal. They may be fascinating, but they aren't helping her get where she wants to go. Perhaps Ellen had set an unattainable goal for herself and this was her way of avoiding failure, or perhaps she had never set a goal at all. Helynn's own goal of becoming an archeologist was unattainable and, like Ellen, she spent too many years at the college smorgasbord devouring classes on impulse rather than by design.

Fortunately for the aspiring student today, there is diversity not only in choices but also in institutions offering courses; everything from auto mechanics to playing the cello to nuclear physics is offered somewhere. Learning times vary from six weeks for a Certified Nurse's Aide candidate to ten years for a postdoctoral student in microbiotics. The cost of a formal education is as varied as the schools and the curricula, but the cost can be minimized. Loans, grants, scholarships, and work-study jobs lessen the financial burden. Once you decide on a goal and map out a course of study you'll find the money is, more often than not, available for the asking. This book will help guide you through what can seem like a confusing maze of options and services.

Socially speaking

If a disabled person is going to strive to do his or her best to live a full, happy, productive existence, a social life is imperative. Living like a hermit in a cave in the Himalayas or in a hut at the edge of the garden like St. Rose of Lima is not exactly a twentieth-century life-style. At least not for the average American. People are by nature gregarious, and even those who are shy need to get out and interact with others.

Start by inviting friends over for a coffee klatsch in the morning or a poker game at night, depending on your disposition toward these activities. Or drop a hint to your best friend that you'd enjoy a "welcome home from the hospital" party. Balloons. A magician. A Highland piper. Anything to help break up the awkward moment that could otherwise grow into a large, leaden silence. A party with a little planning will eliminate that.

It doesn't matter how you start (one-on-one or a dozen at a time), but it is important to begin as soon as possible. The longer the wait, the harder it is to pick up where you left off. Weeks become months and your friends drift away, following their own pursuits. Keep in touch with your old group, if only by telephone. As you grow and develop in your new pursuits, you will meet new people and make new friends who will share your new-found interests. But don't be too hasty about letting go of those who know you as you once were. Whatever happened to you was physical, and that does not—should not—change the person you were into someone different. You need those who share the memories of the past. The past is the basis upon which the future is built; hang onto the best of it, at least.

Depending on the range of the physical handicap, traveling—or simply going out—can sometimes be a logistical challenge akin to Hannibal getting his elephants over the Alps. Bob S. has a severe respiratory problem; he can't breathe without mechanical help. He works in a downtown office. He didn't ever see it as impossible. At night, he sleeps in an iron lung; by day he uses a portable "turtle shell" he plugs into his car cigarette lighter when driving anywhere. At the office, he plugs it into an electrical outlet. There are all sorts of ingenious solutions like that, and we'll point out several similar ones. With some knowledge of what is available, a healthy dollop of imagination, and a sense of adventure, the logistics of movement can be worked out with a minimum of hassle.

Remember that a safe, cozy life of routine and comfort soon goes stale. Without change, without the unexpected, ennui sets in like a gray pall. It happens in an insidious way, creeping silent as a cat into the room. And once life has set itself into a safe, comfortable pattern, it's hard to break away from it. Don't let it happen in the first place.

Organizations to help you cope

Beyond your own social circle, your friends and relatives, you can tap into an endless number of organizations. The foundation that provides practical help (and raises money for research) for people with your particular problem is always a useful contact: get in touch, volunteer, or drop by its office. But make contact. It is true that some local chapters are better able to help you than others; that depends on the dynamics of the staff. But with a mixture of patience (which may be why we're called "patients") and perseverance, you'll find that there is always one person in the office who will be especially helpful.

The people working and volunteering in the many health foundations are knowledgeable about what aid is available, about educational opportunities, and about what careers are open to those in your circumstances. Join, and become a volunteer your-self. You'll learn a great deal, and you'll get the chance to help others.

At the conclusion of this book you'll find the names and addresses of numerous national organizations and agencies which exist to help the disabled. This list is by no means exhaustive, but it can give you a good start on developing your own contacts in a variety of help areas.

Time to take a break

A hobby can be both a pleasant diversion and a catalyst that offers money-making or other sorts of opportunities. People with hobbies form clubs to promote and share information about their favorite pastimes. In fact, there are probably more hobbies than there are people! Surely there is something to pique your interest: stamp collecting, ceramics, chamber music, model-ship building, amateur ("ham") radio, square dancing (with a wheelchair), writing, literature, history, computers. The list is literally endless. Become active in a local group. If you can't get out to meetings, invite the group to meet at your house from time to time. But do it.

A hobby can provide years of creative entertainment. It can furnish you with the opportunity to interact with others on a common ground, one where your physical disability will not be a deterrent. Just be sure the hobby interests you. If (once you've tried it) it doesn't, drop it before you've invested too much time and money. You can choose from plenty of others. Explore the field. Talk to people. Read the magazines. In other words, approach a hobby the way you approach everything else: with a plan.

School presents another resource for social activity. There are strictly social groups such as fraternities and sororities; there are also academic clubs for specific disciplines such as the French club, mathematics club, and archeology club. The athletic teams may be a bit more difficult to be a part of, but look into one or two of them anyway if sports interest you. You could work as a referee, a scorekeeper, a timer, an equipment manager. A campus activity makes going to school more fun (remember, "All work and no play makes Jack a dull boy"). An extracurricular activity adds a bit of zest to college life and should be indulged in on occasion. It's how you meet people and find friends with similar interests.

Finding what's right for you

Probably the most important question you have to ask is "What am I going to do with my life?"

As many different answers to that question exist as there are people who ask it. For some the answer will be clear; for others it will be clouded by doubt and indecision, just as it is for able-bodied people. Often the same quandaries present themselves. Do I really want to do that? Am I really interested in, say, statistics? Enough to spend my life working with them? Is bookkeeping dull? Isn't everybody into computers? If they are, how about the competition? You can lie awake nights pondering such questions, building up indecision and creating doubts like an adolescent seminarian wondering if his call to the priesthood was a true one. Well, unless you *are* contemplating the priesthood, you needn't become bogged down by such intense soul-searching. Relax. You'll come up with something; most of us do.

Beyond the simple need to earn a living, the disabled person should (and needs to) work, for several reasons. Work gives a solid foundation to life and a base on which to build for the future.

More important reasons for having a job exist, of course. One of the most compelling is money. The income of the physically disabled person is chancy at best and almost never adequately covers the necessities of day-to-day living. It seldom includes money for those extra goods and services needed simply to make life bearable. The allotment to pay for the cost of orthopedic appliances, household help, and attendant care is so minimal as to be nonexistent. California has decided (beginning in 1990), for example, that a quadriplegic confined to bed can live on an income of $602 a month—for rent, utilities, food, clothing, doctors, hospitals, medicines (those not covered by Medicare and/or insurance), and personal care. It is an impossibly inadequate sum, and—worse—if you earn any money, the state deducts that amount from your check. Federal, state, and county welfare is available, but in every instance it too is woefully inadequate and shows no signs of getting better. So the need to establish an independent income is a great incentive for embarking on a plan of action leading toward an independent career.

For the young person who has not yet decided on a career or ever held a job, and for the older person who must now make a career change, the quest for the right goal is similar—with the possible exception of the older person who may not have to change to a new discipline but who may find a different career within that discipline. For example, an archeologist who can no longer dig can now do cataloging or set up museum exhibits. An assembly-line worker or an automobile mechanic may have to make a total break with his or her line of work and try something very different. Or that worker may find that another spot on the line will work perfectly or that working as the service manager in the garage is a satisfactory substitute for crawling around under cars. Some will welcome this; others will not. In some cases, where once you went into the workplace to your job, you may find that you must work at home. Such dislocation is difficult but, with persistence, can be managed. The important thing to remember is that, ultimately, the decision to work or not—and where and what kind of work to do—must be thought out carefully and rationally before it is made.

Above all, don't be afraid of mistakes. They can be corrected, and they're a sign of progress. Once you've set your goal, forge ahead—assuming, of course, that you decide on a career. Once you've decided on a course of action, it is best to stick to it. In everything, times of doubt and times of certainty will haunt you. You have to work through the former and hang onto the latter.

Of course, we can't come up with the perfect profession for you. But we can, and will, guide you toward finding what's right for you by suggesting the questions you can ask and the things to keep in mind. We'll also explore several options for working at home.

You can't do it alone

This introduction is just a quick glimpse at the form and substance of this book. The problems identified here are problems all physically disabled people face to one degree or another, and the solutions have been only lightly sketched out. The following chapters will explain in detail how to implement these solutions. Read them carefully. Show them to your family and friends so they can gain a better understanding of your problems. Give them a chance to come up with their own suggestions for assisting you. You're going to need all the help and understanding you can get. Accept it willingly and gratefully. Remember: no one ever does it alone. Sir Edmund Hillary would never have gotten to the top of Mount Everest without Tenzing Norgay and a band of Sherpas. And you won't either.

CHAPTER ONE

Help Is Where You Look for It

When Helynn had polio, thirty other children in her small town also came down with the virus. She was the only one to be paralyzed. The question "Why me?" is unanswerable if you are a victim of birth defects or a disease such as polio. When you awaken some day with a disability, your next task becomes learning to cope with that disability. Your job is to get on with your life.

The first thing to do, once you find yourself disabled, is get over feeling sorry for yourself. This is probably the most corrosively destructive mood anyone can sink into. At one time or another it gets hold of all of us, able-bodied as well as disabled. When it does, all our morbid fears and negativity rise to the surface and can, if we don't watch out, render us all but useless.

When you stop feeling sorry for yourself, stop asking "Why me?" and begin reaching out to others for help, you have begun the first steps toward being in charge of your own life. Sometimes this change from dependency to independence comes so slowly you aren't really aware of it. Day by day you make what may seem unimportant decisions only to discover later that you have actually begun making major decisions about your life. And, with

Empowering the Disabled
BY SUSAN KATZ

Traveling the electronic highways a while back, I ran into a woman named Georgia Griffith. I don't remember exactly the context or the conversation, but someone had left a message on CompuServe asking for help setting up a business for himself. Georgia replied, based on her background as a woman in business for herself.

I continued to see her name occasionally as she interacted with others on the system (she's the "forum administrator" of CompuServe's Handicapped Users' Database, maintaining an electronic database on such issues as devices, sexuality, and parenting). To tell you the truth, I tucked her name under a mental file that probably had the heading "Active and Interesting."

Only two years later did I discover that Georgia Griffith is both deaf and blind.

Using her two computers, a modem, and a piece of equipment called VersaBraille that allows her to read messages, Georgia works from her home in Lancaster, Ohio. She joins thousands of other formerly "disabled" persons across the country who use computers to work and live professional lives not previously possible.

Among Georgia's colleagues: people like Daveed Mandell, a blind journalist in Berkeley, California; Faron Wickey, a quadriplegic software

a rush of exhilaration, you know you are in charge; you have things under control again. For some of us the decision to take charge comes in a blinding flash, and for better or worse we dive right in. But before you can effectively take charge of your life, you need to gain confidence in your ability to make positive choices for yourself.

Counseling

One of the first things to consider is professional psychological counseling. Counselors are trained to help us overcome our feelings of inadequacy, especially the inadequacy brought on when we suddenly find ourselves disabled and, temporarily at least, engineer in Plano, Texas; Craig Werner, a blind English teacher at Buffalo State College (New York); Tony Young, a quadriplegic writer from Washington, D.C.; and Joyce Smith, a blind medical transcriptionist at Wake Medical Center in Raleigh, North Carolina.

Dozens of computer bulletin board systems (BBSs) that concentrate on information and message exchange for the disabled exist around the country. (Several are listed in the appendix.)

Those who frequent these BBSs include people like Mike Bowen, who runs Equal BBS in Raleigh. Bowen, a former bureau chief for the Columbia (South Carolina) *State* newspaper, has multiple sclerosis. It has affected the feeling in his fingers.

"In two days," he says, "I went from ninety words per minute to five." Rough landing for a man who made his living by his hands. While learning how to compensate for the loss of sensation, Bowen became interested in computers as well as issues of the handicapped. He put his three already-written novels into the drawer and took a different tack, creating in the process Equal BBS.

Now Bowen, in addition to running the BBS (gratis), is a computer consultant. His specialty? Training handicapped applicants. (And yes, mystery fans, he does plan to take up novel writing again!)

For any computer user, disabled or not, the possibility of running into people with attitudes like Georgia Griffith and Mike Bowen makes the call to a BBS worthwhile.

© Susan Katz 1987

dependent on others for our care and well-being. They are also trained, obviously, to help us learn to deal with a variety of other issues. In short, counselors can guide us through the trauma of finding ourselves physically disabled in a frightening world where we see ourselves as victims. Locating the right counselor is of prime importance, but it can be a challenging task. You are in uncharted territory—uncharted to you, that is—and need someone who is in possession of a reliable map.

Approach the selection of a counselor as you would approach any other challenge: in an orderly, thoughtful way. Do some reading about family therapy. Virginia Satir's *Peoplemaking* makes a good place to start. Next, talk to your social worker, physical therapist, rabbi or pastor, or physician. Any of them can undoubtedly recommend a counselor who deals with disabilities—

perhaps someone who is also disabled. When you speak to prospective therapists, ask if you can talk to former clients. Also, note how you feel talking to the therapist. Are you comfortable? Do you feel rushed or at ease? Such questions will help you select the counselor who is right for you.

Obviously, becoming disabled changes many things—for you and for your family. That disability may suddenly change the way you fulfill your role as parent, spouse, employer or employee, or whatever. Because of that change, you may experience a sense of loss. The person who has to fill your role, on the other hand, may feel frightened and, sometimes, even angry about having to assume more responsibilities. Most people faced with a situation similar to yours or your family's have had similar feelings. For a discussion of those feelings, take a look at Dr. Elizabeth Kübler-Ross's *On Death and Dying*. It considers such subjects as grief responses and accepting losses and outlines steps you can take to get on with your life.

Remember, re-establishing your emotional well-being is an important step to your recovery. If you don't develop a comfortable rapport with your counselor, look for another one. Once you find a counselor you trust and feel comfortable with, stay with him or her.

In addition, you can learn a great deal by reading. Books like *What Color Is Your Parachute?* and Dr. Bernie Siegal's *Love, Medicine, and Miracles*, and others mentioned throughout this book, can teach you a great deal about how to cope with various aspects of your life. What Dr. Siegal has to say, for example, about illness and the interrelationships of mind and body is applicable to everyone, regardless of the patient or the illness. Several such books are available. Don't overlook them as an important source of information.

Your local bookstore is often the most practical place to start looking for one of the books mentioned here. If it doesn't have or can't order the title you want, you can always order directly from the publisher. Your city library will have a current edition of *Books in Print*, which will give you the book's International Standard Book Number (ISBN), its price, and the publisher, besides the title and author. Another alternative is the *Reader's Catalog*, a listing of more than two hundred categories of books. Orders can be placed through an 800 number. To receive the

Peggy Mellinger

Peggy Mellinger lives by one simple rule: "Don't think negative thoughts—they're destructive."

Although she's been disabled (from polio) since she was twelve years old, she's never asked for, and never expected, anything special or different from life.

"Nobody in my family ever told me I couldn't do anything," she says. "When I came home after the polio, I still had my chores, like everybody else. I guess I was bright enough to figure out a way to do whatever I had to do despite my braces and crutches."

She spent her life—including the time she was getting a degree in business administration from American International College in Massachusetts—in braces and with crutches until an upper-vertebrae condition caused her to change to a wheelchair in 1976. Nevertheless, at fifty-eight, she has raised three children, one a doctoral candidate at the University of California at Santa Barbara. With the children grown, she manages a home for herself and husband Paul in Port Hueneme, California. The house has no special modifications.

"I'm no different from anyone else," she says. "No one is perfect. Everybody has limitations. My limitations happen to be more obvious in other people's minds."

Peggy will still try just about anything, she says. Then she explains that after growing up and living her entire life in western Massachusetts, she and Paul packed and moved to California in 1985 with no place to live and no idea what the future held.

"The important thing is attitude—yours and that of the people around you," she explains. "You have to *try* to do it. Anyone has to try. If you know your limitations, you can always figure out a way to do what you want."

Reader's Catalog, write to them at 250 West 57th St., New York, N.Y. 10107, or phone (212) 333-7900. Ordering instructions and the 800 number are listed on the first page of the catalog.

Finding the motivation

The zest for life has to be self-generated. No magic elixir can engender in you a sense of wanting to be up and doing. You can't just lie in front of the TV and wait for someone to come along and give you the motivation you need to get yourself going.

Motivation comes from within, not from outside ourselves. We aren't all victims of fate; we have the option to motivate ourselves, even when we try to deny it. The surest way to dive into the wave of ambition is to want something. The more you want something, the more motivated you will be. Life is a challenge that is worth accepting. Let ambition stir your blood, and all sorts of exciting things will begin to happen. Once you feel motivated, once ambition and desire come bubbling up, you will be overwhelmed by an invigorating restlessness. When this happens you are ready to begin setting goals.

Goals to guide your life

Much has been written about the so-called midlife crisis, the period when people go through a re-evaluation of their lives. A physical disability brings on the same introspection. Among the things that are irrevocably changed are your long-range goals, as well as all the little ones along the way. Sometimes these need only to be modified to fit your limited physical abilities; other times they have to be changed drastically.

Generally, we tend to resist change. But, stubborn as we are, we have to face up to the reality of our situation and make adjustments accordingly. We must be flexible enough to adapt when the situation calls for it. Just don't ever let go of one goal without having another one to take its place.

Goal modification might have something to do with our professions. If so, take advantage of opportunities for retraining. Remember, a musician can become an arranger and an archeologist can become a museum curator. In any field, a variety of niches is open to those willing to be retrained.

A company called Add-A-Pearl became popular in the 1930s, and the concept still exists. A parent could buy a gold chain with one pearl when a child is born; a pearl can be added at Christmas, on birthdays and other occasions. By the time the child is eighteen she owns a valuable necklace. This same idea of a series of short-range goals leading up to a long-range goal can be applied to travel, education, investments, and the like. And the beauty of it is that, if you are stopped anywhere along the way, you have what you achieved up to that point.

As a brief exercise, jot down a list of things you would like to do with your life (it will be good practice; you'll make several more lists before you finish this book). Don't bother to figure out if any of them are realistic or not. It might be a long list or a short one. Include all the crazy dreams you ever had. Not a bad list, is it? Now divide this list into several smaller ones using headings like "Possible," "Realistic," or "Difficult." Put the paper away for a week and try not to think about it, then do it again. When you're finished, compare the two exercises. What does the result tell you about yourself? Are you consistent in your desires or are you changeable? Did you place your goals in a similar category or are they different enough to be divided among several headings? If you have something listed the first week and not the second, cross it out; also do the reverse.

Now pick an item from the "Realistic" heading and concentrate on achieving it. Start modestly. Just as a pearl can become a necklace, a drive to the next town can become a week in Paris; a class at your community college can evolve into a career in electronics. It isn't too difficult to parlay short-range goals into a long-range one if that is what you want to do, but don't forget that easy, reachable goals can be satisfying enough to be ends in themselves.

Yes, you ARE worth the effort

Eleanor Roosevelt once said, "No one can make you feel inferior without your consent." Call it what you will—self-worth, self-esteem, or self-confidence—it's all the same: a belief in your own importance, a sense that you can determine what shape your life is going to take, that you are in charge of your fate. This feeling of well-being exists in all of us to begin with, but the flame can sometimes burn so low it's in danger of going out. It's natural for us to experience bouts of low self-esteem from time to time, and natural for someone recently disabled to question self-worth. It's the result of the world we live in.

Self-esteem is one of the things you'll deal with in counseling.

Whatever Works for You
BY DIANNE SHIELDS

It's nice to read and hear about people with multiple sclerosis sailing, marathon-running, skiing, and so forth. They should be proud of their accomplishments.

But sometimes these feats can be discouraging to others. You wonder if your family is thinking, Why can't you do more? If he's taught himself to ski, why can't you learn to climb over the back fence when the berries are ripe?

I went sailing with my stepson this summer. He doesn't know it yet, but that was my last time. Some people may say I lack courage; I feel I'm using my head. If for some reason he lays the boat over in the water, I know I'll spend eternity in Davy Jones's Locker.

After the larger-than-life people come the vitamin-and-gluten diets. I'm not knocking them. Whatever works for you is fine.

I read an article about an author who had MS. I tried his plan of massive vitamins and decided he must have a stomach made of iron. Two weeks later, after countless vitamins, all I wanted to do was throw up. It was obvious the plan wasn't working too well for me.

Through trial and error, over the years, I've found a few things that work well for me. All have to do with mental attitude.

The most important is keeping a sense of humor. When the butter dish has just left your hand and it lands upside down—splat—on the

Advertising and society teach us that our worth as people is somehow determined by how we look and what we wear rather than by what's inside us or what we can contribute to our world. One quick way to evaluate your own concept of your self-esteem is to take stock of your attitude. Ask yourself some pointed questions: How do you feel about yourself? Do you like who you are, regardless of your disability? Are you ready to "take on the world"—or are you sullen, convinced that life has dealt you a rotten hand? Your attitude about yourself and life around you will help you identify feelings about yourself.

A quick way to improve your self-esteem is to give it something to feel good about. Tackle—and solve—a problem, any problem. Do that, and you'll notice that your self-esteem has improved kitchen floor, it's a lot better to laugh than to go into the bedroom crying. The minute you laugh, everyone relaxes. What the hell, it can happen to anyone.

The next is finding an interest. My first attack of MS left me sightless at times and at other times I saw more than was actually there. Six months before this attack I discovered the Galloping Gourmet on television. He doesn't know it, but he gave me an interest in cooking that will be with me the rest of my lifetime.

I don't mean to imply I cook all the time. Thank goodness my husband has a taste for canned beans because he occasionally has to fend for himself. He always says, "I've never tasted a bad bean." No one in her right mind would trade a husband with this attitude.

The last item on my list is keeping up your appearance. It takes time but is worth the effort. It's awfully easy to let your appearance go when you don't feel well. It will give your sagging spirit a lift all day to know you look nice.

You don't have to be a runner or athletic ace to feel good about yourself. Above all, surround yourself with happy people. There is nothing like a "Weeping Wilma" to bring your spirits down. There are some people in this world who thrive on being unhappy. You can't bring their spirits up; they only drag yours down. There is no substitute for happy, interesting people. With them and a hearty laugh once in a while, the world will look a whole lot better.

immensely. Periodic doses of success do a lot to improve our concept of ourselves.

Sometimes the issue of mobility, the ability to move about at will, becomes entangled with self-esteem. A physical disability often limits mobility, and our society applauds the ability to move about at will. Others have the ability to move about as they want, and our tendency is to want to be like our peers. Conformity offers a sense of security and a sense that we have succeeded in achieving acceptance. That bolsters our self-esteem. For the disabled, though, the issue comes back to self-pity and the need to remember that the disability is not going to go away. Learning to accept and live with a disability is an important step in building, or rebuilding, self-esteem.

Dave Breslin

Learning to accept and live with a disability can take a long time, especially when the disabled individual is a child. Learning to live with the loss of a limb can take longer.

For Dave Breslin, the acceptance process took more than ten years. Breslin lost his left arm when he was two years old. In a scene he recalls vividly to this day, the arm was caught in a mangle (a type of ironing device with rollers popular in the 1940s).

He recalls that "most of my life, I hid it," even though he doesn't like and doesn't use a prosthesis.

"I was a master at hiding it," he says. "I was so good at hiding it that you could be with me for months and never know. You would *never* be on my left side, for instance."

But something that happened when he was in high school changed that.

"I had a friend I'd met at school," he remembers. "About three weeks after I met him, and after we'd done things together four or

Friends and allowing interests to grow

Friends form an ongoing part of our personal lives. Those who are intimate with our daily lives influence not only the direction our lives take but our thoughts and belief systems as well. For that reason, if for no other, it's important not to shut out friends when the unexpected happens and a disability results.

Yes, the natural tendency is to shut ourselves away from everyone and everything around us in the face of a major medical trauma that leads to a disability. To do that is a temptation we all need to resist. Lasting friendship takes time and effort to build and, once it's established, it is a valuable treasure. One of the most valuable aspects is that a friend doesn't disappear because we look different or because we now move around in a wheelchair instead of "on foot." A friend accepts us completely, doesn't judge us, understands our foibles and flaws. Because of that, although our instinct is to run when disability occurs, we're far five times, I was walking down the hall at school and I was off guard. I heard somebody say 'David, what happened?'"

His friend was shocked.

"He came running down the hall," Dave says. "His face had gone white and drained, because he thought I'd lost my arm between the time he'd met me and that day. I'd maneuvered him so well that he didn't know."

After that, he stopped hiding his disability. He got into sports.

"I was good at sports, and that's where I got my sense of myself," he says. "Baseball, basketball, track, I played 'em all hard and wouldn't give up. That's where I learned not to give up and to be self-reliant."

Now forty-five, Breslin is a librarian at Ventura College, a community college in southern California. He says the best advice he got when he was just out of high school came from a friend who told him, "You have to learn to live with yourself first."

That he's done. He says he stopped thinking of himself as someone different a long time ago.

"If I had both hands, life wouldn't be any different, really," he says. "Except that it would be easier to drive to the left."

---

better off if we allow ourselves to rely on our friends to help us get through the rough times.

We widen our circle of acquaintances by building on shared interests and activities. Joining a club is one way to expand your social circle; the wider the circle, the more apt you are to develop new and like-minded friends. Hobby groups, community college classes, and political-party activities are some more places. Local politics and such organizations as political action committees (nonpartisan organizations working toward a particular goal, like improved benefits for the disabled) are good places to develop like-minded acquaintances who might turn into friends. You'll read about such groups and organizations in your local newspaper. If you find you're interested in getting more involved, take a name from the story and look it up in the phone book. Don't be afraid to call. PACs, especially, are always anxious to find potential members. You'll almost certainly find yourself receiving an invitation to a meeting and on your way into a realm of activity where you can make a positive contribution and find new friends.

Give your doctor credit

Perhaps the most important advice we can offer about doctors goes like this: Don't blame the messenger for the news. It's natural for anyone to feel anger, even rage, when first told that he or she will be unable to walk, or has lost a limb, or has suffered spinal-cord damage. In fact, doctors don't usually expect to see any real progress toward recovery (to the extent that recovery is possible) until the patient's frustration has been worked out. That's one reason why, in the hospital, the newly disabled person is often confronted with a bevy of professionals: doctors and nurses, yes, but also psychologists as well as physical therapists.

The initial tendency in any such scenario is not to trust the doctor's diagnosis, to convince yourself that somehow a mistake has been made and that, as a result, you're going to get well. After that, the next tendency is to blame the doctor. Don't.

Patients tend to view a doctor alternately as a kind of god of healing who brings good health and a long life and as a doomsayer parceling out pain and death. Guard against this, for such concepts distort the truth and make it difficult for you and the doctor to have a realistic relationship. Remember that teamwork and trust are absolutely essential if any sort of progress is going to be made. Without trust, cooperation begins to crumble, and when that happens the chances for success fade.

Don't be afraid to ask your doctor specific or clarifying questions about your circumstances. It's important that you understand every aspect of what the doctor is asking of you. If you don't understand why a particular treatment doesn't seem to be working, discuss it. Perhaps you're expecting results sooner than you should. Perhaps you and your doctor are overlooking something that can help. Perhaps you simply don't understand the medical terminology the doctor uses to describe your situation. Regardless, you should ask. Otherwise, you won't know, and your uncertainty can erode some of your trust in your doctor.

Doctors aren't miracle workers. As a patient—don't think of yourself as a "victim"—you have the right to expect medical progress toward alleviating your distress and improving your health, but you should avoid any temptation to demand a cure when none exists. To do so places doctors in a position from which they cannot extricate themselves. Such overexpectation by patient, family, and friends is common but can seriously endanger the doctor/patient relationship.

The nurse/patient relationship is nearly as important as the doctor/patient relationship. Nurses and patients often form a special kind of bond, especially when the nurse comes into the home. This isn't altogether surprising. The doctor sees a patient infrequently, while the nurse is on hand daily. The nurse, by the very nature of the profession, becomes fully aware of both the illness and the patient. The patient finds compassion at a time when he or she feels helpless, and that compassion is comforting.

The patient, of course, must be aware of his or her dependent situation. The important thing for the patient is to realize that he or she is a "working partner" on this team that is after better health, if you want to make *any* headway against your illness. In other words, take an active role in your own well-being, not a passive one.

How a disability affects the family

Simple day-to-day family living is never really simple under the best of circumstances. When a physical disability has to be dealt with, too, a whole series of crises can crop up. A disability changes the rules of the game for everyone, and new rules have to be worked out to the satisfaction of all the players.

The financial burden that frequently comes with disability is not always the most difficult aspect of that disability to face. Unfortunate as it may be, the changes that involve curtailing the physical activities of a family member are what is often seen as a monumental disaster— because all aspects of family life are affected. The many interrelationships in a family group become strained very quickly in unforeseen ways, and this makes them difficult to deal with.

People are uneasy around a disabled person mainly because they aren't sure what is expected of them. How is a wife supposed

Dealing with the Consequences of Polio and Post-Polio Syndrome

BY DR. PAUL HASAK, Ph.D.

While the following article deals primarily with Post-Polio Syndrome, it can easily apply equally to any degenerative muscular disease. It does not matter to the individual what name the physician gives the disease. What matters is the effect of the illness on the patient's physical body. It is inevitable that a serious set of emotional and mental situations will arise from any serious disability. It is of paramount importance that these be worked through.

Dr. Hasak has condensed these psychological stages into a basic, simple-to-understand approach that is invaluable for your deeper understanding of what is going on in your mind and emotions when you find yourself disabled.

As you read, you will soon realize that you are not alone in these feelings. You are undergoing a perfectly normal human set of reactions to a catastrophic occurrence.

Dr. Hasak, a graduate of Rutgers University with a Ph.D. from the University of Kentucky, is a clinical psychologist who counsels polio survivors at St. John's Rehabilitation Center, 615 South New Ballas Road, St. Louis, Mo.

The issues and concerns identified by individuals dealing with the consequences of polio and post-polio syndrome usually follow from the loss of physical function and the need for change that the loss might entail. The emotional consequences of the physical losses are similar to those seen in the grieving process and include sadness, anger, guilt, fear and feelings of being alone in the world. The intensity of these mixed emotions can at first be quite overwhelming and result in a state of "shock" whereby the emotional system shuts down or at least leaves one in a state of confusion or depression. If the emotions are allowed expression their intensity lessens over time. However, whereas the grieving process may be understandable and acceptable in the loss of a loved one, it is often not considered acceptable for other types of losses. Adjusting to the loss then becomes more difficult as you attempt to deny or avoid what you might consider "unacceptable emotions."

Changes that may be required as a consequence of loss of physical function can affect every aspect of your life—family, work roles, responsibilities, as well as your self-image. Guilt, shame and self-criticism often follow for not being able to "overcome" the symptoms. Overcoming rather than adjusting to realistic limitations is possibly in your history as an individual who had to deal with the consequences of polio. "No one knew I had polio" was the accomplishment. Now it may be more difficult to hide or overcome the physical deficits and you somehow interpret this to mean that all past efforts have been in vain and that you are a failure. Loss of confidence and reduced self-esteem soon follow. Being unacceptable to yourself, you often fear and attempt to avoid rejection from others by withdrawing.

A sense of control and security usually accompanies having established an acceptable routine and style of living. This is threatened by the need for change. Fear of an uncertain future is increased by imagining the worst possibilities; for example, "I will be a vegetable, useless to myself or to anyone and totally dependent." Dependency on crutches, a wheelchair, or others is a change that conflicts directly with longstanding beliefs in self-sufficiency and independence.

Denial and avoidance may seem like the only way of coping. These, in fact, might be helpful early on when you are overwhelmed by the thoughts, emotions, and consequences you are facing. Adjustment begins when you are able to examine all of the emotional reactions un-self-critically. It is then possible to begin looking at the meanings you are attaching to your situation and which are producing your particular emotional reactions. Given our tendency to overgeneralize in our thinking when we are feeling something very strongly, some of the meanings might be unrealistic and incorrect and can be changed.

Support groups can be an excellent way of beginning to deal with these psychological and emotional consequences. These groups can provide an opportunity for giving permission to feel the feelings you are having. They also allow the benefit of being understood and accepted at a time when you are feeling most alone and frightened. Finally, groups can provide an opportunity to acquire information and learn how others are dealing with their situations. Individual counseling is also available to aid in identifying the unique meanings you are attaching to your situation at a time when emotions are high and interfere with the ability to maintain focus and objectivity. Even though you might be able to get through it on your own, the support and resources available could help shorten the length of time it takes and perhaps even ease some of the pain of the struggle.

to react to a paralyzed husband? How should a child feel toward a helpless mother?

To make matters worse, the paralyzed husband or mother doesn't really know how to react to the able-bodied members of the family. Drawing up a workable road map is doubly difficult because each person involved is emotionally unique. The same problem can befall a dozen different families and, since each family member is an individual, the dozen different families will respond to the crisis in their own ways.

Once again, this is where counseling, either by a professional or by a member of the clergy, can be of inestimable help. There's no doubt that the situation is complicated. A counselor can help untangle all those threads of strained emotion and raw nerves. Most important, remember that the right family response can be worked out with a bit of love and understanding. If the family was a happy one before the crisis of disability, it can regain that happiness and go on to explore new and different avenues.

CHAPTER TWO

Independent Living

Independence simply means choosing your own life-style: where and how you will live and the direction in which you will pursue your own brand of happiness. It means learning to rely on yourself to solve problems, and it means learning to live with your disability and within its limitations. It also means making your own way in the world. How we do this is up to us. What and when we do it depends on all sorts of factors—financial and physical among them—and perhaps a bit of luck.

This entire book is about independent living; this chapter contains a variety of tips and guidelines that have worked for others. In the following pages we will try to sketch out various scenarios—not with any intention of telling you what to do, but in the hope of outlining options open to you. Every one of us lives according to daily decisions that we are constantly making. Most of these are so small or insignificant we don't consciously think about them. Nevertheless, over the years, our lives are built upon them. One of those decisions involves the degree of independence we want to establish. For some of us, the extent of our disability may help tip the scale in one direction or another.

Jim Ritter
BY SHARON WHITLEY

What happened to Jim Ritter graphically illustrates the need for independent living.

"My main concern for people disabled from accidents is that— no matter how old they are—their mothers tend to baby them," says Ritter, thirty, who was paralyzed from the neck down in an accident. "When someone in the family gets hurt, it's usually the mother who takes care of them.

"My accident happened when I was sixteen and my mom babied me until I was twenty-three, when she died," he says.

Jim counsels parents to act as if the person isn't handicapped.

"If you treat them as handicapped, they're going to be handicapped," he says. For six years after his accident, Jim depended on his mother. "She did everything for me, and at age twenty-two I was still thinking like a sixteen-year-old."

When his mother died, he suddenly had to learn to be on his own.

"She hadn't explained a thing about Social Security to me, or anything else," he recalls. "Mothers try to overcompensate for the disabled person, but they really need to help them to be more independent."

Ritter suddenly found himself having to care for himself.

"When Mom died, I moved in with my brother," he says. "One day my sister-in-law said, 'Today you're going to sit in a wheelchair.' At first I resented it because they were making me work, but now I realize that it was the best thing that could have happened to me."

Prior to that, he had had no social life, he says.

"People at church would invite me places where I'd have to get in the wheelchair," he remembers. "They'd say, 'Let's go to the park,' and if I wanted to go with them, I'd have to get in the chair. Within three weeks I couldn't wait to get in my chair and go somewhere."

Jim counts himself lucky that he's always had family support.

"After I lived with my brother for nine months, he decided it was time for me to be on my own," he recalls. "I finished my A.A. degree and am now working on my bachelor's in art. I've had a lot of obstacles along the way—a little bit of everything. But I've always had a need for independence."

Regardless, each of us, able-bodied or disabled, has his own concept of independence.

When it comes to financing an independent living situation, the able-bodied and disabled face the same set of budgetary issues: housing, utilities, food, transportation, insurance, clothes, entertainment. But the disabled frequently have one extra expense: a personal care attendant. Making it all work out budgetarily can seem like juggling Jell-O at times. But with a bit of compromise here and there you can usually come up with a budget that will work.

Paying your own way

Of course, the biggest problem we all face, disabled or not, is making enough money to meet our expenses and have a bit left over to put away for a "rainy day." It's unfortunate that, too often these days, there just doesn't seem to be enough to go around. Still, several things you can do will save you a few dollars here and there. Taken all together, those savings can add up to quite a lot in a short time.

First, before you move into an apartment, condominium, or house in any city, contact the utility company or companies. Explain your physical situation; some utility companies reduce their rates for customers who have to operate life support systems such as respiratory devices or who need extra heat for medical reasons. It never hurts to find out what special programs might be available.

Next, call your phone company's office that deals with the needs of the disabled. You probably won't get a reduction on your bill here, but this office can supply you with specialized phones. In California, Pacific Bell sends a technician to your home to determine what phone will best meet your specific needs. This evaluation is free; so is the phone. Be sure to inquire about a similar service in your area of the country *before* you move into a new place so it can be installed early and ready for use. Incidentally, if you already have this service at your present home, think about how long it's been since you asked for an update. New telephone gadgetry (like one-button dialing and even voice-activated dialing) is rapidly coming on line. Don't shortchange yourself if there's something that can make your life better.

If you were able to work twenty of the past forty quarters and paid into the Social Security fund during that time, you may be eligible for Social Security benefits under the disability program. Contact your local Social Security office for information. If you do qualify, be sure to follow all instructions to the letter. For more detailed information write for the excellent brochure on Social Security benefits to the Nebraska Polio Survivors Association, P.O. Box 37139, Omaha, Neb. 68137.

Government agencies—federal, state, and local—are continually changing their monetary assistance to the disabled, and many of us do not get all the benefits we're entitled to because we often don't know what they are. Obviously, it's important for us to be informed when a change occurs; unfortunately, getting the information is seldom easy. You generally have to dig for it. Your social worker (assigned to you when you first applied for Social Security or other aid) will be able to give you leads. Follow every one of them diligently, even though it can become tedious. It could mean extra money to live on.

For whatever reason, very few people or agencies volunteer any sort of information; you usually have to ask for it directly. Even then it isn't easy. But if you look at the process as detective work or a treasure-hunting expedition, it will be less frustrating. Don't get discouraged. Funds are out there to help you, but the amounts and qualifications vary from state to state. Be persistent, and you'll unearth what you're entitled to. Until the implementation of a uniform federal criterion for aiding the disabled, we're just going to have to cope with a hodgepodge of regulations and pay scales.

Whether you're going to be living on your own or sharing with family or friends, there are many ways to enjoy the good things in life and avoid going into debt to do it. You can, for instance, go to the movies early in the day—most theaters have lower "early-bird" rates. Restaurants usually charge less at lunch than at dinner, and some also have "early-bird" deals; the food is just as good and the ambience the same. No matter what, always remem-

---

Tips for Calling Government Offices

First, always call early in the morning (no later than 10:00 A.M.), no matter what the office. Government agencies never have enough people to answer the phones, and those they do have get busier (and their tempers get shorter) as the day wears on.

Second, write down your questions ahead of time and try to anticipate what the person you talk to will need to know about you—age, degree of disability, employment status, or whatever. Being prepared will facilitate your call and will save wasted time making follow-up calls that could have been avoided.

Sometimes you're required to send in your question in writing. If this is the case, be sure you find out the proper office—the agency may have more than one location. Helynn once wrote to the main Social Security office in her city and received no answer. Several weeks later, she wrote again and asked why no one had answered. This time she got a phone call telling her the first letter should have gone to her neighborhood office. The main office would not forward the letter! Nor would she have learned of her mistake had she not written again to demand a reply.

---

ber you're not poor; you're just a bit low on funds. Poverty is a state of mind, not a state of checkbook.

Personal care attendants

Choosing a personal care attendant (PCA) is every bit as important as finances, career, and education. In many ways, your relationship with your personal care attendant can be like a marriage—your PCA is a caregiver, a friend, a helpmate, and often a pair of able hands. Hiring—and keeping—a PCA can be difficult and frustrating. It can also be fabulously rewarding.

A job that is as difficult as housework, involves looking after the physical needs of the disabled, *and* pays minimum wage seldom attracts the upwardly mobile section of society. Fortunately, those who choose this profession seek greater rewards in life than financial gain. More often than not, you'll realize before long that your PCA is more than just a helpful, interesting good companion. He or she often becomes your best friend.

When you seriously consider hiring a personal care attendant you need to identify several things. Make two lists. On one, list what you can do for yourself; on the other, list what the PCA will have to do. Be totally honest in these appraisals. You might want to feel you can do certain things without help, but the fact of the matter may be that doing them exhausts you unnecessarily. Don't gamble your health. If you feel you may need help sometimes, add those times to the PCA's list. Overconfidence in what you can physically accomplish daily can lead to medical as well as practical problems. And you don't want to add to the job description *after* you've hired someone.

After you've made your lists, use them to develop a job description. Be completely fair to people who read your advertisement. Outline job duties, whether you need round-the-clock or part-time assistance, and list wages. From the very beginning, before you start interviewing applicants, be clear about what is and what isn't expected. Although everyone understands that some modifications may need to be made from time to time, neither you nor your PCA wants to be confronted with a barrage of the unexpected.

If you need to hire a nurse to come to your home on some sort of regular schedule, you should have a rough idea of the classifications of nurses. The most costly, by virtue of extensive medical training, is the registered nurse. An RN administers medicines, takes samples, changes dressings, and checks vital signs.

Licensed vocational nurses (LVNs) are often underestimated, but make no mistake: their training is excellent and they are, as a group, highly competent. They are also a bit less expensive than RNs.

The certified nursing assistant (CNA) is a trained individual capable of doing the less medically demanding nursing chores. The period of training is short, generally only a few months, but is adequate when illness is no longer in the acute stage. The CNA is instructed in the general care of the patient but is also a housekeeper.

If you need continuous care, your best bet may be to hire a

full-time, live-in helper. It is less expensive than employing three people for eight-hour shifts and much less disruptive. But a live-in PCA must be given time off each week for personal recreation, shopping, visiting, theater, sports, or whatever. Don't ever expect anyone to work without sufficient personal time. It's unrealistic. When your PCA is off, family members and friends are usually willing to fill in, or a local volunteer agency dealing with your disability might be able to provide someone.

To get the best information about ways to finance your PCA, ask your welfare worker what is available in your community. This varies significantly from state to state and county to county, but it is safe to say that funds are out there. In some cases, the state pays the PCA directly; in others the money is sent to the disabled person and he or she pays the attendant.

A word to the wise: if the money comes to you for disbursement, make it clear that your PCA, as a self-employed worker, is solely responsible for his or her own taxes. Keep a record of whom you pay and the amounts for your own future protection.

You can advertise for a PCA any number of ways, depending on your needs. The local branch of the organization that provides assistance to people with your disability may be the best place to start. Hospice is another possibility, since it maintains lists of volunteers routinely. If you're fortunate enough to live near a medical or nursing school, the placement office there can also be an excellent resource. Churches and their newsletters can sometimes be helpful, too. Still another alternative might be a classified ad in one of the magazines for the disabled. Although you'd attract a large pool of local applicants, we counsel caution about classified ads in local newspapers since you don't know what kind of people you'd be hearing from. You might also consider the local unemployment office.

One suggestion: Many single-parent women are looking for a place to live for themselves and a child. A place to live and a small income at a job where she can be home with her child may be an attractive opportunity for such a parent. For you, a child around the house can be a delight.

When you begin interviewing possible PCAs, pay close attention to these things:

- Appearance, both grooming and dress. You pay attention to your appearance; you have a right to expect the same from an employee.
- Speech. You want someone who's articulate and interesting to talk to, especially if this person is going to be around twenty-four hours a day.
- Attitude toward life in general and you in particular. We're not all "upbeat" all the time, but someone interviewing for a job should be presenting his or her best self, and you're looking for someone with a positive approach to life.
- Common interests and preferences. If you're going to spend a significant amount of time with this person, it's important for you to know how your likes and dislikes match up. If you're a sports fan and your attendant doesn't know a baseball from a tennis ball, you may run into a communication wall. Find out his or her idea of a good meal or an enjoyable movie.
- Training credentials. Find out if the applicant has earned a job training certificate.
- Previous experience and references. You should ask whether he or she has worked in this field before. If so, ask why he/she is changing jobs. Then check references. References aren't always wholly reliable, but you'll sometimes get added information the applicant didn't give you.

Finally, don't hire on the first interview. Ask each applicant to call you at a certain time. Whether they do will tell you how badly they want the job, whether they tend to follow through, and if they're punctual and attentive.

We've only sketched a few ideas for hiring a personal care attendant. Some booklets and at least one full-length book are available on the subject. If you're in any way still hesitant about hiring a PCA, you might want to consult one of the sources listed on this page.

Food

Along with rent and personal care attendant's salary, food is a costly item in anyone's budget. There may be several ways you can

Finding a PCA

More and more people with physical limitations are using help from personal care attendants (PCAs). *Home Health Aides: How to Manage the People Who Help You* is a handbook to teach people who use PCAs how to find, train, manage, and pay these workers while keeping them happy.

As the spinal-cord injured quadriplegic user of a motorized wheelchair, author Alfred DeGraff has hired and managed PCAs in various settings: college campuses, career offices, urban apartments, rural homes, and health facilities.

The more than eighty-five topics in this book include settings for using help, strategies of a good manager, factors of good work environments, types of needs that do and do not qualify for help, ways to request help, making a list of needs, creating a job description, sources and methods for recruiting, interviewing and screening, hiring and training, and using agency aides versus personally recruited help. The book sells for $18.95 (plus $2 postage and handling) from Saratoga Access Publications, Box 2346, Clifton Park, N.Y. 12065.

The Independent Living Research Utilization (ILRU) project offers a set of three booklets collectively titled *Independent Living with Attendant Care*. The first, "A Guide for the Person with a Disability," is a twenty-page booklet that focuses on finding and hiring personal care attendants. The twenty-four-page "A Guide for the Personal Care Attendant" is aimed at those looking for employment as PCAs and covers concepts of disability and independent living. The third booklet, "A Message to Parents of Handicapped Youth," is a twelve-page publication that discusses teaching independent living techniques and responsibilities to children and advises on when to use PCAs.

These booklets, written in 1980, are $3.50 per booklet or $10 per set and can be ordered from ILRU, P.O. Box 20095, Houston, Tex. 77225, or 3233 Weslayan, Suite 100, Houston, Tex. 77027.

deal with this. Try for food stamps. Whether you are eligible or not depends mainly on your income, and several restrictions apply. If you qualify, the stamps cost a percentage of their face value—they're a real bargain. If you don't have a cook (or even if you do and want to allow some time off), the Meals on Wheels program is a great option. Meals on Wheels is a volunteer program that operates virtually nationwide (look under *Meals on Wheels* in the phone book). For a very reasonable flat monthly fee, the people at Meals on Wheels deliver to your home every noon (except weekends) a full hot meal and a cold one for supper. This ensures you of a balanced daily diet each week. It's an excellent and helpful arrangement for disabled and the elderly who find it impossible to shop and cook for themselves.

Another way to help bring down food costs is to join a food co-operative. Like everything else, these co-ops have variations in their rules, but the basic object is clearly the same: cut down on food bills by wholesale cooperative buying. For instance, a group might charge $12.50 plus four hours of your time bagging groceries for, say, an equivalent of $35 worth of food. For those in the co-op who are unable by age or disability to give four hours of work, that requirement is waived. The only thing that could be viewed as a drawback is that you generally can't choose what vegetables you want because co-ops buy what's in season or what is surplus to keep the cost down. In all, a co-operative can be a good deal for you and the other members, too. Look in the Yellow Pages for an entry like "Cooperative Store" under "Grocers." Call and ask to have rules for membership mailed to you.

Finding a place to live

A large part of independent living means living in your own place, rather than with relatives or friends. One of the biggest challenges— and at the same time, one of the greatest adventures— for the disabled person involves finding a place to live.

Before you start looking for a place to lease, list your priorities. Consider the following in determining what you need:

- Number of bedrooms. One for you, one for your personal care attendant if he/she is with you around the clock. Remember, a small bedroom can serve as an office if you're going to work out of your home.

Independent Living Resources

Two national organizations that help with resources for independent living for the disabled are the Independent Living Research Utilization Project (P.O. Box 20095, Houston, Tex. 77225 Phone: [713] 797-0200) and the National Council of Independent Living Programs (c/o Max Starkloff, President, 4397 Laclede Ave., St. Louis, Mo. 63108. Phone: [314] 531-3050).

The ILRU Project is a national resource center for independent living. It produces resource materials, develops and conducts training programs on independent living issues, provides technical assistance and consultation to independent living centers, and publishes a monthly newsletter that addresses matters affecting the independent living field.

Its major resource is the *Directory of Independent Living Programs*, which lists programs and the services provided by each on a state-by-state basis ($8.50 prepaid). Individuals are invited to contact ILRU for free referral to projects near their communities and to write for a complete publication list.

NCILP is a professional association for member centers, disseminating information about independent living matters and relevant legislation through its membership network. It can provide referral to a local program to consumers, up-to-date practical information to professionals, and advice to persons interested in starting an independent living center.

◆ You may have to overcome stairs to get in the front door. Find out if you can install a ramp if you promise to remove it when you leave; most landlords will readily agree.

◆ Size of the living room. This can be important if you need an assistive device nearby which takes up a lot of space. Helynn's living room needs to be large, for instance, because of her iron lung.

◆ Other available space. This depends on what you're planning to do besides live here. If you plan to make craft items to sell, for instance, you might need a larger-than-normal kitchen area or an outdoor patio to do this work.

◆ Width of hallways and door openings. Make sure your

wheelchair will fit. You don't want to discover *after* you signed the lease that you can't get into the bathroom!

◆ Adequate electrical outlets. Many older places don't have enough, and you don't want to be strapped for a place to plug in, say, a computer and a respirator at the same time.

◆ Note the noise in apartments around you. Loud radios or screaming children may not bother you, but you may want to think about the noise level before you decide.

◆ Determine whether stove and refrigerator come with the place. Don't let yourself in for a sudden expense.

◆ If the place is not on the ground floor, be certain you're comfortable with the elevator, especially if you're completely unable to manage stairs.

◆ Check the neighborhood. Does it appear clean? Sedate? Do residents seem relaxed? Friendly?

These are just a few things you might include on your checklist. Put down everything that is important to you so that you don't forget something vital. Check these things out before you sign the lease. After you complete your list, read Marene Aulger's home design section in Chapter 5. It might remind you of something you've forgotten, and it will certainly give you a look at what can be done to make things easier for yourself.

As usual, money is a primary concern. Living on your own can be a risky financial step, and you want to minimize that risk as much as possible, for your own peace of mind if nothing else. When you go out looking for a place to live, you need a lump sum of cash on hand—large enough for a cleaning deposit and your first and last month's rent if you're renting or large enough for a down payment if you're buying. In addition, the advice that you should always have enough saved to cover two months of general living expenses is sound. A bit of a nest egg like that will give you a feeling of security and relieve some of the anxiety you'll experience during the early stages of your venture.

"What can I afford?" is normally the first question you need to ask yourself. Of course, we're assuming income from some source—a job, an annuity, or government assistance—but we all have to live somewhere. At one time, economists agreed that one-fourth of your income was a workable amount to pay for shelter. These days, if we go by that formula, it probably won't be enough. The high cost of housing is a fact of life that none of us can avoid. You can take advantage of three elements, however, that work to your advantage: patience, friends, and rent control.

First, avoid falling in love with the first place you see. Be patient. Keep looking, and don't be afraid to tell real estate agents or prospective landlords what your budget limit is. Occasionally you'll find that the rent can be lowered a bit to come within your budget. The property owner probably has a mortgage payment to meet, and that payment comes due whether the place is rented or not. Rental income makes the payment, so it's to the owner's advantage to keep the place rented. Another tip to keep in mind: it's sometimes possible to trade services for an allowance against the rent. If the owner has a gardener come in once a week to cut the lawn and trim shrubs, for instance, you and your personal care attendant might be able to trade those duties for reduced rent.

Time and your friends are on your side when you're househunting. You can dragoon an army of friends to act as advance scouts. You just may come up with an affordable gem. Your friends can scour the town for you as they go about their normal activities, and you can do the follow-up calling.

Rent control limits the amount of rent that can be charged in normally high-rent areas. Areas of Los Angeles and New York fall into this category, for example. When someone moves, the rent can be adjusted upward, but frequently you'll stumble across a centrally located delight at a remarkably affordable price. Ask a realtor about rent-controlled areas and keep inquiring about availability of places in those areas.

Buying a condominium or a house is certainly better than renting because the place is *yours*; *you* get the advantage of the property's increase in value, and you can make any alterations you want. You also get the responsibility of fixing things that go wrong. Be sure to bear that in mind when you consider buying. If you decide you'd prefer to fix it yourself (or pay to have it fixed) rather than call a landlord (as you would if you were renting), fine. Just make sure you consider that aspect.

If you buy a condominium, make sure you can live with the

covenants and other restrictions. Some can be so restrictive concerning additions or structural changes that you might not be allowed to build a wheelchair ramp to your door or install a lift track in your bathroom ceiling (many California housing developments even specify the colors houses may be *painted*). A condo does have many advantages for a disabled person—gardeners and maintenance, for instance, as well as clubhouse and pool—but the restrictions can be troublesome. Check them out before you buy.

A house may or may not have as many covenants as a condo, depending on where it is. Older homes usually are freer of restrictions than newer developments. Normally, though, aside from concern for architectural integrity, you can pretty well do what you want.

Whatever you do, don't give up. Eventually you'll find the right place, whether you rent or buy. If you find a house or an apartment that is in the right location and has what you want but is larger than you need, consider sharing it with someone. Sharing living quarters is one way to cut down on expenses and many people do it. If your place is near a college campus, for instance, you can almost certainly rent a room to a student easily. Caution: It is better to sign the rental agreement yourself and sublet to your partner. That way it's *your* place; if you and your renter/roommate don't get along, you are the one who stays. Also, make sure you have your landlord's permission to sublet.

When Wilma, Helynn's personal care attendant, said she wanted to go to San Diego State University for a degree in art history, Helynn suggested they move near the campus. Everyone else said, "You'll never find a place. Thirty thousand students are desperately looking for apartments in that area." In only one afternoon of knocking on doors, Helynn and Wilma found a place close enough for Wilma to walk to classes and still within their rental budget. After Wilma graduated, Helynn said, "Now we'll move to La Jolla and live on the beach." Again everyone said, "You'll never find a place you can afford; only rich people live there." After an afternoon of knocking on doors, they found a cottage. That night Helynn fell asleep listening to the sound of the surf pounding on the sandy beach. It isn't all luck, although that helps, too. But Helynn and Wilma found places by identifying the area in which they wanted to live, by setting aside the time to find a place, and by making the effort. They did it, and you can, too.

Getting out and around

How to get from here to there has always been a big problem for the disabled. In past centuries, the wealthy were carried about in sedan chairs on the shoulders of footmen.

It was only two hundred years ago that a wicker bath chair with wheels was devised for use at European health spas. By contrast, today's wheelchair is a true miracle of human ingenuity. A wheelchair will do just about everything you want it to and take you almost any place you want to go. Self-powered, electric-powered, wheels, tractor treads, pontoons, heavy, light, rigid, folding, large, small, whatever you can imagine can be obtained (see Chapter 5 for complete details). About the only drawback to all of these marvelous advances is that the cost of transportation is, like everything else, high. Do a lot of shopping around before you buy anything. You'll find, if you keep in touch with local hospital supply stores (or anywhere else wheelchairs are sold), that there is a steady turnover in wheelchairs. Users often upgrade, so you stand an excellent chance of picking up a previously owned chair at big savings.

You should shop for a car in the same cautious way. Look for easy usability and comfort. Keep economy in mind. Figure into the cost any modifications you'll need to have made—lift, controls, whatever. Various manufacturers offer special deals for the disabled from time to time; ask about any such incentives (such as free installation of hand controls, for instance) at your local dealership. Bear in mind that having a car will cost you money, sometimes whether you drive it or not; garage rental can be expensive, too. See Chapter 5 for detailed information about lifts, racks, and hand controls.

Public transportation is a slightly different matter. Here you have to deal with bureaucratic regulations that, until recently, have not always been sympathetic to your requirements. Meanwhile, by nature public transportation is often, at best, difficult for the

Mobility Equipment

A number of firms specialize in adapting various vehicles for use by persons with mobility impairments; and several are listed here to get you started. Their services may include installation of lifts, custom controls for hands or feet, power doors, or other modifications. Often, existing family vehicles can be adapted, although sometimes purchase of a different vehicle is necessary. Used vehicles are sometimes available through classified ads in periodicals aimed at persons with disabilities.

In all cases, consumers should contact a variety of sources and compare prices, quality, and warranties.

♦ *Braun Corp.* For the dealer nearest you, phone 1-800-843-5438.
♦ *Howard Burkett, The Rincon Corp.,* 11684 Tuxford St., Sun Valley, Calif. 91352.
♦ *Cameron Enns Co.,* P.O. Box 5019, Fresno, Calif. 93755. Phone: (209) 222-2922.
♦ *Drive-Master,* 16A Andrews Dr., West Paterson, N.J. 07424. Phone: (201) 785-2204.
♦ *Freewheel Vans, Inc.,* 4901 Ward Rd., Wheat Ridge, Colo. 80033. Phone: (303) 467-9981.
♦ *Gresham Driving Aids, Inc.,* P.O. Box 405, Wixom, Mich. 48096. Phone: 1-800-521-8930.

disabled to use. American subways (indeed, subways around the world) generally provide an accessibility challenge that is difficult to surmount, although you can with patience and persistence.

City bus services, on the other hand, are required by federal law to be wheelchair-accessible, although you might encounter some reluctance to comply in some communities. If you encounter difficulties in your city, contact the political action committee that is working on such problems.

You should also get in touch with any taxi companies operating in your city and ask about their policy toward the wheelchair-disabled. You'll probably need to use a taxi at one time or another, so the prudent thing to do is to check out all the nearby companies ahead of time. In some places, you can call a Chair

- *Handicapped Driving Aids of Michigan, Inc.*, 4020 Second St., Wayne, Mich. 48184. Phone: (313) 595-4400.
- *Handicaps, Inc.* 4335 So. Santa Fe Dr., Englewood, Colo. 80110. Phone: (303) 781-2062.
- *Kroepke Kontrols*, 104 Hawkins St., Bronx, N.Y. 10464. Phone: (212) 885-1100.
- *New Era Transportation, Inc.*, 810 Moe Dr., Akron, Ohio. Phone: (216) 633-1118 or 1-800-325-9649.
- *Haveco*, 421 Amity Rd., Harrisburg, Pa. 17111. Phone: 1-800-692-7293 (Pennsylvania only) or (717) 238-1530.
- *Mednet, Inc.*, 544-546 WaWeeNork Dr., Battle Creek, Mich. 49016-0948. Phone: (616) 962-3800.
- *Mobility Products and Design, Inc.*, 3200 Harbor Lane, Minneapolis, Minn. 55441.
- *Tri-State Mobility Equipment Co.*, 940 Cleveland Ave. S.W., Canton, Ohio 44707. Phone: (216) 489-6666.
- *Vartanian Industries, Inc.*, P.O. Box 636, Switzgable Dr., Brodheadsville, Pa. 18322. Phone: (717) 992-5700 or (212) 863-7043.
- *Wells-Engberg Co.*, P.O. Box 6388, Rockford, Ill. 61125. Phone: 1-800-642-3628.
- *OTHER SOURCES:* Check with the Center for Independent Living nearest you for assistance and suggestions. Also, a book on this subject, *Going Places in Your Own Vehicle*, is available for $6.50 (plus $0.70 shipping) from Accent Special Publications, P.O. Box 700, Bloomington, Ill. 61702.

There organization in advance if you need transportation to someplace like the doctor or a civic event. This specialized service usually carries a small fee because it is operated by a nonprofit group. The organization that helps people with your disability should be in a position to tell you about the availability of this service in your city.

Canine Companions for Independence (CCI) is a nonprofit, tax-exempt organization founded in 1975. CCI trains specially bred dogs to assist people with disabilities other than blindness to live independent lives.

Service dogs aid people with orthopedic challenges; *signal* dogs alert the hearing-impaired and deaf to crucial sounds; *social* dogs are placed with individuals or in institutions as part of pet-facilitated therapy; and *specialty* dogs are trained for seniors or individuals with multiple disabilities.

CCI executive offices are located at P.O. Box 446, Santa Rosa, Calif. 95402-0446. Phone: (707) 528-0830 (Voice/TDD).

Sexuality and relationships

Most of us daydream about sex as though it were a fast-tempo game of musical chairs, with us whirling around to the music, spinning with the captivating sounds and lights and smiling faces of our brief partners. But sooner or later the game ends. That's when it's nice to have someone to go home to.

Contrary to the ads on TV, sex is not everything. The able-bodied and the disabled alike often fall into this trap, but the disabled sometimes fall into a far more subtle snare: they fall in love with their PCA. It's easy to understand how and why this happens. The PCA is the person who provides comfort, safety, compassion (which is often mistaken for love), and encouragement, all things we want in a PCA to begin with. It becomes hard to resist those strong feelings. The problems begin, of course, when you meet the "significant other" of your PCA and find your feelings shattered. The long-term effects on your relationship with your PCA can be endangered. On the other hand, your attendant might share your feelings. There have been cases in which such an occurrence has grown into a rewarding life-long relationship. The best way to avoid a painful situation later on is to discuss your feelings openly with your attendant and find out if those feelings are reciprocated.

In this era of AIDS, it is not only prudent to limit your sexual partners, it is vital. Nor is exposure to AIDS the only risk you take. No one is entirely safe, of course, but you can't let this panic you into a monastic state; you need, however, to show a bit of common sense and maturity in your sexual activities.

However, Bill Bowness, a disabled counselor, notes that the main problem when you're wheelchair-bound is dating and how to meet people. "When I did sexual counseling, my clients weren't nearly so worried about sex as they were about finding dates. I'd tell them to get out and do things. Join an art class, take an interest in a sports team, go on a picnic. Be where people are relaxed, doing things. Don't worry about dating per se. Just take part in life."

Some people in wheelchairs find they have the most success dating people who have some previous awareness about disability. "All of the women I dated were working with the physically disabled in some way," Mike McIntyre explains. Mike recently married the rehab nurse he dated. "I knew she understood my problems," says Mike, "so I felt more comfortable." Naturally, one type of person who is familiar with wheelchairs is another person in a wheelchair. Don't overlook this possibility, for companionship.

No matter what life-style you choose to lead, "living together" is not the same as "living happily ever after." Keep in mind that you have a far better chance of succeeding in any kind of long-term relationship if you are attuned to the notion that the need for periodic separation is not rejection.

If you are married to a nondisabled person, you may have doubts about whether you can have sex at all, whether it will be different, or whether you can be a parent. Probably the most important thing both you and your partner can do is be completely honest with one another in discussing your questions and feelings. Both of you should discuss issues you can't resolve with your counselor or with your doctor—perhaps both. Remember that technological advances are coming along almost daily. In recent years, for example, the development of prosthetic devices have allowed men formerly unable to have sex to function normally. Options like these, plus honesty with your partner, can help dispel fears about marriage or other long-term relationships.

If you are hiring someone to help with the chores, hire a personal care attendant rather than a housekeeper. Constant, twenty-four-hour attention is too much togetherness for anyone. There can be too much of every good thing, even chocolate and love. A staleness can set into the relationship that can seriously endanger it. Both of you need regular separation time, however brief. Even if it's something as regimented as a separate "night out" once a week, it can breathe vitality into a relationship.

Aid to Adopt Special Kids
BY SHARON WHITLEY

Two people who have never let a child's physical characteristics get in the way are Bob and Dorothy DeBolt, the founders of AASK. Throughout the years, they have adopted fourteen children "with special needs." Basically, these children need a family "who can love you, push you when you need it, help you do your best," said one adopted handicapped child.

The family's economic stability is not as crucial to adoption agencies any more, Bob points out.

"The financial aspect should be the second or even third item considered in adopting a child," he says. "But if there are going to be major expenses with the child, we have to look at community support."

The DeBolt family consists of Korean-Americans, blacks, Vietnamese, and Caucasian children with all kinds of special needs: some are blind, some don't have legs or arms, some can't walk.

Today all the DeBolt children are on their own—Sunee, of Korean descent and paralyzed from polio, is married and gave birth to a healthy baby girl in 1988. Sunee teaches piano and is active in her church, where she sings in the choir.

The other children are equally successful. Tich, a paraplegic who

So you want children

If you and your spouse really want children, you have as good a chance medically and physically as anyone else. Yes, some able-bodied people are unable to conceive or carry a baby to term, and the same is true of the disabled. Some people just cannot have children, but until you exhaust every avenue open to you, there is no reason for you to give up. Medicines exist today to help; so do prostheses for the disabled male. Thanks to medical science, such things as erection dysfunction can safely be corrected. Most important: don't be discouraged by short-term lack of success. A negative attitude can be a depressant that guarantees more failure.

When you consider having children, your doctor is a vital ally.

was wounded in Vietnam, has a bachelor's degree in computer science. He lives with Anh (who also has a degree in computer science) in an apartment in Berkeley (which they share with sister Ly). J. R. (John Robert)—who is blind and a spina bifida patient—lives with a blind roommate in Oakland and plans a career as a paralegal. Karen, born without arms or legs, now lives by herself in Oakland and attends junior college.

Since 1973, AASK has placed over 5,000 special-needs children. The organization now has offices in twenty-seven cities throughout the United States.

"We have a rate of over 90 percent successful adoptions," says Bob. "We created an organization to find and help families willing to adopt physically and/or mentally handicapped children of all races in need of permanent homes. The role of AASK is to change the public awareness of who's adoptable and who isn't."

Potential adoptive parents find out about AASK through word of mouth, the documentary films that have been made about the DeBolt family (*Who Are the DeBolts and Where Did They Get 19 Kids?* with Henry Winkler and *Stepping Out: The DeBolts Grow Up* with Kris Kristofferson), parent support groups, or adoption groups. AASK has no adoption agency fees.

"We look at the parenting skills of an adoptive parent—not their age or color or even economic situation," notes Bob. "We have placed kids with disabled singles and couples."

He or she can advise you of any potential physical problems, of course, as well as whatever other factors you might need to bear in mind, like possible difficulties nursing or dressing an infant. With the expertise and cooperation of the right doctor and regular monitoring, your chances of having a child are excellent. But, if you are unable to have children of your own, seriously consider adoption. Information on adoption by the disabled is presented below.

Don't for a moment consider that you can't raise children if you're disabled. Peggy Mellinger, who has been in a wheelchair most of her adult life, had and raised three children after she contracted polio. Helynn cared for her nephew, Larry, for periods up to a year even though she was confined to a bed. In short, it can be done. Just bear this in mind: parenting knows no disabilities.

Adoption as an alternative

If you long for a child to complete your family and can not have one of your own, consider adoption. It can be done. One of the first places you should contact is AASK (Aid to Adopt Special Kids), 450 Sansome St., Suite 210; San Francisco, Calif. 94111, Phone: (415) 434-2275, which handles the adoption of disabled children. Getting in touch with them can change your life, as interviewer Sharon Whitley learned.

Until a few years ago, county adoption requirements were very strict: almost always the only people able to adopt a baby or small child were middle- or upper-middle-class couples. Adoption agencies tried to "match" the couple to the child in race and other physical characteristics. Children with physical or mental handicaps were typically overlooked and left to live out their lives in hospitals or orphanages. And couples with physical disabilities never had a chance to adopt a child.

But now all that is changing. Because of a variety of social changes in the past twenty years, fewer babies have come up for adoption. Older children are now being adopted by single parents, disabled parents, parents with economic hardship. No longer is the criterion the perfect middle-class home.

In the words of the shoe company, "Just do it!"

The longer you delay your entrance into the mainstream of society, the more difficult it gets. If you've read this far, you don't want to withdraw into your own world. So resolve to fling open the doors.

Start your blazing social whirl by inviting a few relatives and friends in for an hour or two in the afternoon for soft drinks or tea. If the weather is good, have a backyard cookout. Try an evening of cards. Sometimes just a friend and a chess game can be heady stuff. But build a network of acquaintants. Several good places for socializing are community-sponsored activities at your local recreation center, church functions, special school activities, and holiday events such as picnics and dances.

Regardless, hiding in a dark Victorian environment isn't going to do it. Whether you're in a hospital, at your family home, or on your own, you can find ways to enlarge your circle of friends and to enjoy an independent social life. Be open to new people, new ideas, new situations; get out of your everyday environment whenever you have a chance. If you want a better, "livelier" life, it's up to you to work for it.

CHAPTER THREE

Education: The Best Medicine

One of the questions most often asked on a college campus is "What am I doing here?" The answer most professors give is that today more people in America have college degrees than ever before. That's unquestionably true. But think for a moment about what that assertion means. The vast majority of applicants in today's job market have college degrees. So the Great Job Chase becomes just that much tougher a contest for everyone. It also means that if you have a degree, all other things being equal, you (or anyone else, disabled or not) enter the game at least even with the competition. If you and another applicant are equal in ability, qualifications, and other relevant areas, doesn't it make sense for an employer to choose the one who has the college education over the one who doesn't?

You've no doubt heard people say that probably the most important thing anyone can do in life is get the best education possible. Such advice is doubly true for the physically disabled. The reason is simple: your disability is enough of a limitation. Today, if you lack education too, you simply won't have much chance of landing the job you want. Thankfully, plenty of options are open to the disabled person. Take advantage of them, and you're on your way to the career you want.

First things first

If you're still in high school—or if you never completed high school—and you're disabled, the notion of college might seem like a faraway dream. Nothing could be further from the truth. Tiresome as it may sound, there's no time like the present to start planning for the future, and a college education is a vital part of your future. The only difference is that you may have some work to do first to get yourself ready.

Federal law requires that services for the disabled be available in every public primary, middle, and secondary school. And, generally speaking, private and religious schools have followed the lead of public schools, as long as the student can keep up with the regular curriculum. The Education for All Handicapped Children Act of 1975 says that no one may be refused an education solely on the basis of disability. Public schools that fail to comply risk loss of federal funding. This law means two things: first, if you're in high school now (or any other level, for that matter), you have a right to the services and accessibility you need to obtain that education. Second, you can expect to be mainstreamed. Private schools are usually open to accommodating the physically disabled, but sometimes don't have the funding that public schools do.

Bureaucratic as the word may sound, *mainstreaming* simply refers to integrating disabled students into classes with nondisabled students. As a result, you may have to take greater care to avoid becoming lost in the shuffle. So this is the time to learn an important lesson: you're going to have to ask for, even insist on, the things you need to get the education the law says you're entitled to. Whether it's testing to identify learning disabilities or getting an access ramp for your wheelchair, don't expect someone else to foresee the need and provide it. Learn to ask for it.

Here are a just a few of the services that must be provided by public schools (at all levels) if you need them: transportation to and from school, speech therapists, sign-language interpreters, rehabilitation services. The list goes on and on. For instance, the Carl Perkins Act makes federal vocational funds available to high schools for vocational training and career awareness classes for the disabled. Services for the disabled will vary from school to school, generally depending on how supportive of special programs the particular district happens to be and how insistent parents are that quality programs for the disabled be maintained. Note, too, that regulations governing private schools may vary considerably from state to state; check with your state's department of education for information. But the bottom line is that whatever you need must be available to you.

Suppose, then, that you're high school age and physically unable to leave home to attend school. What can you do? First, telephone the principal yourself and ask for a meeting to discuss what arrangements can be made for you to "attend" classes from home. Perhaps a computer link can be set up which will enable you to complete assignments and transmit them electronically; or perhaps a special tutor can be hired to sit in on classes for you and bring you up to date daily. Whatever you need, don't be afraid to ask. Doing so will ultimately get the results you're after—an education—and help you learn an important lesson you'll use often in life: how to ask for and get what you need.

America's public schools have endured a great deal of criticism in recent years, some of it deserved and some not. Regardless, the fact is that classrooms are crowded and teachers and administrators may be only vaguely familiar with the special needs of the disabled. This means that while the services you need are available (because the law requires that they be there), you may have to search for them. The easiest way to do that is to meet with your counselor every week. Let him or her know how you're doing in your classes and, above all, whether you need any special assistance. If you're having trouble in a particular area, such as reading, ask about testing. If the counselor is reticent, ask your parents to arrange a meeting immediately. If that doesn't bring results, contact the principal. You're entitled to that assistance, and you're going to need it. Make sure you get it.

All state laws mandate some number of years of formal education, and most four-year colleges and universities want evidence that you've completed high school before they'll admit you. But even if you don't have a high school diploma now—perhaps you left school some years ago because of your disability or for some other reason—chances are you can get one in a comparatively short time. Two popular avenues exist for people to complete high school in later years:

- Adult education
- The GED (General Education Diploma)

Adult education classes are flourishing across America. They are designed specifically for people returning to complete high school, so you'll find a camaraderie there. Classes meet at night and, occasionally, on Saturday. They are generally free.

Is adult education for you? To find out, make a short list. Ask the following questions, and write in the answers:

1. How many courses do you need to graduate?
2. What are they?
3. Are they offered every semester in your adult education program?
4. How many courses can you realistically take each semester?
5. How much time are you willing to spend to get the diploma?
6. How does the time factor relate to the other goals you've established?

One drawback of adult education is that progress is usually slow. While regular high school students may take six or seven classes a semester during the day, adult education students will probably take only four. If you need just a few classes, that shouldn't be a problem. But if a disability has kept you out of, say, your junior and senior years, you could be facing a longer time period than you're willing to spend—perhaps three years, even if you go to school every night. After you've considered your situation and goals, talk to your local district's adult education director before making a decision.

The **GED,** as it is commonly known (the actual name may vary depending on the state), is the other alternative to completing high school. It's attractive to many people simply because it takes less time. You just take (and pass) a comprehensive examination covering material you need to know to graduate from high school. GED exams are given at regular intervals; you can contact your local county's superintendent of schools for a schedule. Classes designed to help you "brush up" and get ready for the test are offered regularly, too. Not every state offers a GED or something similar, though more and more are adding it every year. A call to the county superintendent of schools will tell you whether your state does. If so, this alternative deserves strong consideration because it may be the quickest way to prepare yourself for the next major adventure you're going to face—college.

Campus life: The challenge and the joy

There is more than one reason for going to college because there is more than one reason for acquiring an education. Most students today (as has always been the case) go to school to get a good start, one that will give them upward mobility in their chosen careers. Their choice of university is often of paramount importance: Harvard for business, Massachusetts Institute of Technology for science, the University of California at San Diego for marine biology. Others go to school to give themselves a general education, to broaden their knowledge and to enhance their mental horizons. Some even go for the social activities or the sports opportunities. Whatever the reason, higher education enriches your life, and that is reason enough.

If you're going to college for the first time, or back to school after having been away for several years, a community college (sometimes called a junior college) may well be your best bet. There are several practical reasons for this choice:

1. Admission requirements
2. Proximity
3. Low cost

Community colleges typically have an open enrollment (or admission) policy. You won't have to worry about whether your grades from high school are good enough to gain admittance. As a general rule, anyone over eighteen can go to a community college regardless of prior education. In other words, just about anyone can get in; staying in, however, is another matter.

Remember another important practical consideration: A community college is just what its name says; it serves a localized area, or community. Consequently, you'll usually find a community college within a few miles of home, especially if you live in a metropolitan area. Such proximity is important. Four-year colleges and universities may be more distant—perhaps far enough away that you'd have to (or want to) move closer to campus to make getting to class easier. Moving is an undesirable hassle under the best of conditions. Who needs it? Keep this adventure as simple as possible: as long as it meets your needs, select the school closest to your home. It will pay real dividends in time and frustration saved. Besides, you'll soon have enough to do to keep you busy.

One other feature makes the community college a preferred choice: its comparatively low cost. Few community colleges offer free tuition these days (California's did until 1983 but now charge $50 for a full course load—still mere pennies compared with tuition at state-supported universities). You can be certain, wherever you live, that you'll pay less at a community college. Don't worry unnecessarily, however. Lower tuition does not mean you'll get a "watered-down" education. To the contrary, many of higher education's best teachers, fed up with the "publish or perish" syndrome that has gripped many of the nation's universities for the past twenty years, have moved to community colleges so they can concentrate on doing what they are trained to do: be excellent teachers. Remember, too, the old saying that you get out of any experience what you're willing to put into it. A teacher, particularly a college-level teacher, is there to guide you and to help you think—not to do your thinking for you. A little effort on your part will make even the dullest course valuable.

Besides what are called "general education" courses—those

required for a degree in your state—you'll find a wide variety of majors (areas of concentration) at a community college, just as you would at its four-year counterpart. Often you'll find even more extensive offerings. At the university or four-year college, the primary emphasis focuses on completing the bachelor's degree. The community college doesn't ignore this aspect of education; thousands of college graduates spent their first two years at the lower-cost community college. But community colleges go beyond that. They operate on the philosophy that roughly equal numbers of students plan to transfer to a four-year school to earn a bachelor's degree, train (or retrain) for a particular job, or take a two-year associate degree and go into the job market (an associate degree in commercial art, for example, can be the beginning of a career in advertising or children's-book illustrating). Hence, at a community college you'll certainly find the "traditional" programs like business, the humanities, math and science, and social science. But you'll also find programs in automotive technology, hotel and restaurant management, electronics, even air conditioning and refrigeration.

You'll also find many more courses taught at night than at many universities. Community colleges have long since realized that most people have to work while going to school and that most jobs require an employee's presence during the day. These schools have adjusted their schedules to accommodate a greater number of people in what is generally the most flexible time period of the day. In fact, hundreds of people work full time and still carry a full schedule of classes at night.

Even if you're not working yet, the extensive night schedule can make life easier for you, too. Let's say you want to take a history class, and you have a choice between one that meets for fifty minutes three mornings a week and a night class that meets for two and a half hours once a week. In most cases, it probably makes sense to take the night class. If you're only taking one or two classes, the night class requires only one trip to campus; the morning class takes three. If you're paying an attendant to accompany you to class, it is a less expensive proposition to go one night a week rather than three mornings. So your favorite television show is on that night. You can always catch up during summer reruns or tape it on your video cassette recorder and watch it after you get home.

Besides the advantages of proximity and lower fees at community colleges, two other important factors make these institutions attractive to disabled students. First, states regularly allocate money to community colleges specifically for "pilot" (experimental) programs for the disabled—programs that often don't exist at four-year schools. For example, money for computer-aided instruction for disabled students is being awarded with ever greater frequency. Such assistance programs mean more resources to help pave the way toward your degree.

Second, but no less significant, is the fact that community college physical plants are usually (though not always) smaller and therefore easier to navigate. It may not sound important now, but wait in a few lines at registration. That can wear down even the hardiest constitution. If you've been in a line to register and a line to pay fees and a line for a parking permit, the last thing you'll want to face is a long trek across campus to the bookstore, where you'll wait in line some more. You can't escape the lines, but at least the bookstore isn't as far away on a smaller campus.

If the foregoing seems like an ad for community colleges, it is. Community colleges can provide many of the advantages of a four-year school, they're usually closer to home, and they seem to get more federal funds to assist the disabled than four-year schools do. But they have one disadvantage: their offerings are more limited. If you've set your sights on a bachelor's degree or higher, you might find a community college handy the first two years. After that, you'll have to attend a four-year school. Or, if you're in an area of the country with few community colleges, you'll attend a four-year school from the beginning.

Regardless, everything we've discussed about community colleges applies equally to four-year schools. Laws governing disabled access are the same, for instance. For the rest of it, from bachelor's degree through doctorate, the issue is what you know and how well you apply it. Thousands of disabled students graduate from universities every year and go on to graduate school. The research component inherent in graduate study can, for a disabled person, provide an area in which to excel.

Helynn's Education

Here's how Helynn describes her experiences with education:

My own education was an unplanned patchwork quilt. Not the best way to approach any venture as important as education, but it was the only way open to me. And, in the final analysis, it worked out just fine.

A great many circumstances worked against me, but I was determined to get as good an education as possible for someone with my devastatingly severe handicap. Perhaps it was *in spite* of my polio rather than *because* of it that I succeeded in getting what I wanted.

I went back to school less than a year after having polio. I entered the third grade in March, while I was still confined to a reclining wheelchair. During my grammar and high school days, I was never physically able to attend a complete semester of classes, but I did fulfill all homework and examinations.

We lived in a small town with no special provisions in the school system for a disabled student. To this day, I am convinced that this worked to my advantage, because it taught me how to integrate into the mainstream immediately. The teachers and students helped by pushing my chair, opening my books, putting the pencil in my hand, and they all did it with a willingness that kept me at ease.

Going to college was another problem altogether. There were none in town and my family couldn't afford to send me away to school. I searched about and discovered that the University of Chicago had college credit courses by correspondence. I began my

School with a nontraditional twist

Suppose your goals don't include (or require) a rigorous educational program. Maybe what you want to do just requires one or two courses. Or perhaps getting to a campus on a regular basis is for some reason impractical. What then? Don't worry. You still have plenty of options available.

One of the most appealing is what colleges often call "community service," or continuing education, courses. These are shortened study of Egyptology and was on my way toward my goal of becoming an archeologist.

After moving to Honolulu, I studied Polynesian language and ethnology in University of Hawaii classes taught at the local YWCA. I also took art lessons at the Academy of Fine Art. All of this was sporadic because, by this time, I was working as the first woman sports writer in a wheelchair in the islands, and I was feeling extra pressure to prove myself.

The family next moved to California, where I enrolled in correspondence courses in literature and political science. By then, I realized it was necessary to change my major—physically, I would never be able to fulfill my dream of going on an archeological dig.

Since there are some courses which can't be done by correspondence, I did my laboratory science requirements at Southwestern, a very good local community college, and had the reports sent to the University of California at Berkeley, where I was registered as a student.

I never applied for grants from institutions or for any monetary aid from the government; for some reason or another, it never occurred to me to do so. This absence of money caused innumerable delays in my progress towards a degree. If I were to do it over, I would ask for help from every quarter.

My journey through the field of education, from grammar school to high school to college, was charted bit by bit according to what was available at the time. I was determined to take advantage of whatever was at hand to not worry about the next stage. It took a bit longer this way, but I did get what I wanted—an education that has enhanced my life.

courses taught away from campus. They generally meet in church social halls or classrooms at neighborhood elementary schools. Their duration is short—one dealing with real estate appraising may meet for five consecutive Wednesday nights from 7:00 to 9:00 P.M., while another, dealing with cake decorating, may wrap up after one four-hour session on a Saturday. Occasionally a two-day course will be held on a Saturday and Sunday. Fees vary for these courses depending on what kinds of materials are required.

The subject matter of the courses runs the gamut—from hang gliding to emergency-room nursing to writing poetry and most things in between. Practical skills like calligraphy and desktop publishing are among the popular continuing-education-type courses offered, but the range is endless. The drawback is that these courses rarely, if ever, offer regular college credit (although some offer what are called continuing education units, or CEUs, for people who require regular recertification in a job). But, credit or not, if you're looking for something less traditional in education or for training in a very specific area, this may be the place to look. Simply call your local community college or university and ask for the continuing education office. The names may vary, so don't be surprised if you get transferred a time or two. Eventually you'll wind up with the person you want. Ask for a catalog of current course offerings (they aren't always published with the college's regular class schedule), and you're on your way.

Learning by mail

Another popular avenue, and one that supports long-distance study, is the correspondence course. A special "extension" office on a university campus usually coordinates correspondence courses. Community colleges rarely offer them. That doesn't matter, though, because correspondence courses make it possible to actually come within a few credits of completing a bachelor's degree without ever leaving your living room.

Contact the nearest university extension office for a catalog and look through the offerings. You'll find an array of traditional and nontraditional courses, from political science to creative writing. To sign up for one or more courses (a limit is sometimes imposed by the sponsoring institution), just fill out the form, enclose a check, and drop the package in the mail. Within a week or two, you'll receive a course outline that will tell you how many lessons are involved in the course and what the instructor's requirements are (pay careful attention to these, because they vary considerably from course to course). The outline will also tell you what textbooks, if any, are required. If you can't find the book locally, the sponsoring university's bookstore will ship it to you.

Correspondence courses are self-paced. It's a good idea to discipline yourself to complete and mail in one lesson every week. Most schools allow one year to complete a correspondence course, but if you work at a regular pace for, say, two hours every morning, you'll be surprised at how much you can accomplish in a short time. You'll read a printed "lecture" in a workbook provided by the school, then complete a series of assignments. Type (or have someone type) all your assignments. Then simply mail them to the instructor. The instructor will read and grade your work, then mail it back to you. The first assignment in nearly every correspondence course involves writing a short auto-biography so that the instructor can get to know you. Most of the courses require a final examination; you'll have to have someone from a nearby school (principal, dean, or an instructor), or perhaps a notary public, monitor your final exam and sign and mail it in for grading. It's that simple. The trick to taking correspondence courses is to work at them a little at a time every day. Waiting until eleven months have passed to get started can prove disastrous.

You may not be able to complete a bachelor's degree by mail, but you can take a major step toward that degree. A combination of correspondence courses and on-campus attendance can be a practical way to minimize some of the logistics hassle and still put together a course of study that will lead to a degree. Correspondence-course catalogs will indicate which courses are transferable, but you're well advised to arrange that in advance with your local school. That way you won't run into sudden surprises come graduation time. Required laboratory work can usually be done at the local community college and the credit transferred to the university from which you are taking correspondence courses but, again, make arrangements to transfer the courses in advance.

Similar to the correspondence course but generally part of the school's main curriculum is the telecourse. Most colleges and universities these days offer one or more courses taught using what is known as a residential cable television channel. Other school systems use microwave links to provide such courses to the distant reaches of their service areas. The result is the same: you stay at home, tune in the television at a specified time, and watch the lecture. As with a correspondence course, you mail in your assignments, and the instructor grades and returns them to you. Some telecourses require that you attend a lecture in person once a week or once a month. Others have no such requirement.

Whatever the requirement, telecourses are another option worth investigating. Unfortunately, no central clearing house exists to let people know which schools offer which courses and when. This is partly because each department at a college usually offers only one telecourse a term. The instructor will normally teach the one telecourse (in addition to his/her traditional courses), then step aside to let a colleague have a turn. This means that the course offerings change every semester (or quarter, in some instances), and the college frequently doesn't know until the prior semester what will be offered by television.

An interesting variation on the telecourse concept is Mind Extension University, a nationwide system of telecourses operated by cable television proprietors. The cable operators contract with a school in their service area for a particular course that is then shared among a network of cable systems throughout the country. The idea has great potential in the years ahead; for now, though, be sure to check on credit transferability before enrolling to make sure a course will be accepted in your program.

The best bet for telecourse information: call the office of the vice president of instruction (sometimes called the vice president of academic affairs) at your local college and ask to be put on the mailing list for telecourse information. You might also call the campus television station and ask for a copy of their program guide. Be sure to let them know you're interested in telecourses.

The computer age has opened new doors for learning at all levels. Technological advances have made possible ways of storing, retrieving, and communicating information that were only fantasies a few years ago. Many of these advances have already taken root. The concept of electronic mail—sending and receiving mail via computer—is one small example. The growing presence of computers in kindergarten classrooms is another.

If you have a computer at home, you might as well take advantage of its capabilities. If you don't have one, start a campaign to get one. It isn't a luxury anymore; it's a necessity. Even if you don't plan to earn a degree, a computer will expand your horizons so much that at times the walls of your room will disappear. But you might find that you can earn a college degree right from the keyboard—without ever leaving the room. It's just one more example of how computers are changing our lives.

The Electronic University Network, founded in 1983, can link your computer to more than 100 courses at colleges and universities from coast to coast. In 1989 fifteen schools were participating in EUN, and the list includes some of higher education's leaders: Boston University, Oklahoma State University, Penn State University, the University of Maryland, the University of Iowa, the University of Illinois, John F. Kennedy University, Thomas A. Edison University in New Jersey, and the University of the State of New York. The last three schools offer associate's (two-year undergraduate), bachelor's, and master's degrees.

This intriguing option requires that you have a computer with a device called a modem (you can buy one for as little as fifty dollars—see Chapter 6), which you connect to your telephone, and the software (program) required to operate the modem. Through the keyboard, you instruct your computer to call EUN, and—presto! —you're in class in minutes. It's even possible to ask questions of the instructor on-line. The advantages for the disabled individual are obvious.

The first time you look at the course fees in the EUN catalog, your reaction will probably be that the price is too high. Tuition isn't cheap—a three-credit general psychology or American history course can cost $390. But when you figure the cost of transportation to a traditional campus, along with parking and attendant wages, then add that to tuition and allow something for the time and hassle, you'll find the price isn't as high as you first thought. Besides, when you enroll, EUN sends you the necessary course notebook (which contains a course syllabus, exam information, and related information), the software you need for your computer, and the textbook (which is billed separately). You also gain access to an electronic library that can connect you to a range of research databases. And don't forget, even if you don't have a scholarship to help you pay the cost, you probably qualify for a guaranteed student loan.

Courses you take electronically, through EUN or other programs like it that are sure to follow, are generally transferable to a local college or university, but you should check first to make sure; many schools will transfer your courses but require you to take four or five courses—especially courses requiring laboratory work—on their campus. EUN will provide you course descriptions, accreditation reports, test scores (most electronic courses use standardized final exams), and any other information you may need to give your home institution.

Another electronic college, called Connected Education, is offered through New York's New School for Social Research. It currently offers a master of arts degree in technology and society as well as a certificate in electronic publishing. Connected Education plans a master's in business administration and a doctorate in technology studies before long.

You can order the EUN course catalog, which gives details of offerings, fees, services, and transferability, by sending a check for five dollars to Electronic University Network, 1150 Sansome St., San Francisco, Calif. 94111. The toll-free EUN telephone number is 1-800-225-3276 (1-800-445-3276 in California). For more information about Connected Education, write to Paul Levinson, President, Connected Education, No. 61, 92 Van Cortlandt Park South, Bronx, N.Y. 10463, or phone (212) 549-6509.

Business, vocational, and trade schools

Suppose you decide that a complete college program leading to a degree just isn't for you. Perhaps you want to do something that doesn't require a degree—bookkeeping, for instance. Then what? Do you just take a bookkeeping course and hang out a shingle?

Not really. If you decide this route suits you best, you might be better off contacting one of the business, vocational, or trade schools in your area. A word of caution, however: look for one that has been in business for a long time—it wouldn't stay that way if it didn't have a reputation for graduating people trained in the most current techniques and with sound job skills. To check more specifically on a particular school, though, ask for a copy of its most recent accreditation report (an accrediting agency is a body which certifies that a school is teaching the things it should teach in various disciplines). Ask for the names of some of the school's graduates and talk with them. Ask them about the school, its curriculum, and its teachers. Was the placement office helpful in finding them jobs? Can you get around the school buildings easily? Such questions are important; they help minimize unpleasant experiences. If you are concerned about a business, trade, or vocational school's reputation, call your local Better Business Bureau and ask if any complaints have been filed about the school. Be wary of new institutions boasting grand plans. You have your own plans, and you don't have time to be a guinea pig for someone else's. Besides, it's always possible that the "grand plans" include the director sunning on a faraway beach using your tuition money.

Local trade, business, or vocational schools offer one particularly significant advantage—especially if they are well established: they provide a rich source of contacts for jobs or for clients. Tuition and fees vary greatly, depending on the programs and the number of courses required in each. Costs will nearly always exceed community college expenses but fall below university and four-year college costs. Certification is typically granted upon completion of a program.

Finding the finances

Once you've made the decision to strike out in pursuit of some form of higher education, one of your biggest concerns will probably be money. Financing an education isn't cheap these days, by any standard. But you needn't worry excessively. Literally bushels of dollars await the applicant willing to search a bit and wade through a morass of paperwork.

Some states, for example, provide health care for the disabled while they're in school. To find out, check with the local division of your state's health and welfare (or some similar name) department. Some county governments provide scholarships for the disabled. These often require a written application and a personal interview (they generally just want to meet the person they're giving their money to). There are two ways to find out if your county (or city) government offers scholarships for disabled students: call the financial aid office of the largest college or university nearest you or contact the county board of supervisors. In the first instance, the larger the school, the greater the chances that the financial aid office has dealt with situations somewhat similar to yours and will know the ropes. In the second case, remember that city or county council members usually pay little attention to obscure, less politically motivating programs such as the one you're asking about. Persevere. Be persistent. Don't let anyone put you off until you have exhausted every angle you can think of. Remember: it's your future on the line.

There's another place to look for financial assistance: on campus. All colleges offer scholarship money given by private citizens or corporations. Many of these carry restrictions for applicants regarding major, minimum grades (which must be documented), financial need, or other factors. However, about an equal number are more general in terms of requirements. One California community college, for example, offers a memorial scholarship to "a second-year journalism student who is transferring to a university." No mention of grades is made. Another scholarship at the same school is given annually to the special education department's "outstanding hearing impaired student." The list is virtually endless. You can find out about what is available in two ways. First, a quick call to the special education department should result in a short list of scholarships and grants for which you're eligible to apply. Second, if for some reason you don't get what you want from the first source, call the financial aid director or one of the assistants (you may have to be persistent to get past the secretary) and request a copy of their current list of scholarships and requirements. It's best to have a name when you call that office. Otherwise, because of the constant whirl of activity, you may find your patience with the secretary wearing thin. How do you find out a name or two? Easy. When you phone, call the main switchboard (it's the main number listed in the phone book). Ask the person who answers for the name of the financial aid director and his or her chief assistant.

There. Now you have two names. The operator will connect you. Explain your situation briefly and tell the director (or assistant) that you're looking for scholarship or other financial help to return to school. Remember that word *other*. It can open an entirely new door of financial assistance.

So many different kinds of outright grants, on-campus jobs to earn money, and loans are available through every college financial aid office that it would be impossible to mention all but a few. Just one hint: save the loans as a last resort, to be used only if all other options fail. Schools across America and in many foreign countries offer special direct grants (through federal or state programs, usually) to economically disadvantaged, minority, and disabled students. Certain programs in California, for example, provide for tuition waivers at community colleges. Other grants go directly to the campus bookstore in your name, and books and supplies you need are charged against that credit. Depending on your personal financial situation, financial aid grants to help you pay transportation costs to and from school might be available, and some states have programs that provide a minimum amount of money for basic living expenses. Ask the financial aid officer for a list of grants for which you might be eligible. And ask the special education counselors to help you complete and file the forms the first time. That will help you learn anything you need to know when applying for aid.

Abuse of some of these programs in recent years has caused a tightening of requirements, but the money is still available to people who are willing to apply for it. Some additional advice about grants is in order here: adherence to regulations and politeness are always noticed. Meet deadlines promptly and with a smile. Such an approach is a help in getting more aid later.

Another source of income is a job on campus. Don't flinch. You won't get rich, but you'll be in a less "pressured" environment with people more aware of the restrictions you face. Example: a professor in the English department where you answer the phone twenty hours a week will not complain or threaten to fire you if you ask for a day off to study for an exam; nor will that professor complain if you need to adjust your schedule to accommodate your new class schedule at midyear. The people on a

---

A Sample of Services

What's available to help you at your local college? Here's a short sampling:

- Note-takers for sight-impaired students.
- Specially trained tutors and translators for hearing-impaired students.
- Special classes for students with a wide range of physical and learning disabilities.
- At some schools, limited transportation for disabled students.
- Special (though limited) libraries.
- Trained counselors. (In fact, a disabled veteran will often have the benefit of *two* counselors: a special education counselor and the campus veteran affairs counselor.)
- In many cases, the special education department will even take care of registration for you.
- You rarely have to pay for more than normal tuition and books.

---

college campus know why you're there; they *expect* education to be your first priority. You don't always find that attitude in the workplace.

What kinds of jobs can you do? Whatever you feel capable of. There are dozens of student hourly jobs available: shelving books in the library, answering department phones, typing, tutoring. One hearing-impaired student at Oxnard College in California earned extra money during his second year as a part-time photographer for the school's public relations office. It all depends on your physical abilities. Going to school can be physically exhausting. If so, work only as a last resort. Always keep in mind why you're in school in the first place.

Let them know you're there

Let's assume you've contacted the school's financial aid office, applied for and received a scholarship or other form of assistance from the school, and been admitted to the college. Before registering for classes, there is at least one other thing you need to do.

Be sure to drop by the special education office and meet the people who work there. They are equipped to provide an incredible range of services, available for the asking. Meet with the special education director if possible, or with an assistant at the very least. Explain your situation as completely as possible. Be optimistic but not overconfident. Above all, be completely honest. Don't let the person you talk to think you can do more, or endure more, than you realistically can. That will come back to haunt you.

Your campus's special education office can become a resource that opens doors you might not have thought even existed. If a professor or counselor has suggested that you need specific kinds of education-related tests (motor skills, dyslexia, and so forth), your special education office can take care of them for you—free. You'd pay a lot of money to have a private psychometrist or doctor administer those same tests. The list of services to the disabled provided by these offices is extensive. But don't expect all these services to simply come your way. As with anything else, you won't find answers unless you ask. People won't know what you need unless you tell them.

Keeping it all in perspective

So you've looked through a stack of catalogs and made the decision. There are still a few things to keep in mind. One is to keep your course load at a reasonable level. The average college student will take fifteen units, or hours. Nine or twelve might be more reasonable for you, at least until you get your feet wet. Remember, taking one or two fewer classes means that much more time to work harder for the ones you are taking. It's better in the long run to begin with fewer courses for two reasons. First, your energy level and general physical condition can suffer if you're overambitious. This can, in turn, require you to curtail many of your activities. Second, if you're not accustomed to "cracking the books," you might find yourself becoming bored or frustrated with your stumbling academic achievement. Give yourself the best possible chance to succeed. Start out slowly at first and build up your workload as you progress.

The temptation to take every course in sight and to "window shop" by adding and dropping a variety of courses during the first week of the term is strong. Fight it. Stick to your original plan, the one you and your adviser worked out before you registered.

Make sure that during the first week you find out where the school's academic improvement center (or learning center, or whatever it happens to be called) is located. That's where you'll have the best chance of finding help fast when you need it; that's where tutors are located and where additional resources for specific classes are stored. The center is usually tucked away in the library somewhere. Become a regular visitor. Hire a tutor if you begin to feel overwhelmed by a particular course. The special education department may even be able to provide you with one free of charge; it depends on the school. Meet your instructors after class or during their office hours and ask questions about parts of the lecture you found unclear.

A college campus is a place where a special kind of exuberance exists. It is a vibrant place where students can be found in the cafeteria or coffee shop arguing the philosophies of Descartes and Spinoza, discussing the nature of imploding "black holes" in space, or complaining about something as mundane as the high cost of a parking permit. It's an important part of that unique ambience known as a "college." Take part in those discussions. You'll learn a lot and meet many interesting people.

A variety of organizations exist, too, for people with similar interests. Hang around the student center long enough, and someone will attempt to entice you into a particular organization— that much is certain. Extracurricular activities like this are as much a part of the college experience as formal classes, but you have to be cautious. Again, the temptation to become involved in a variety of activities is strong. All seem worthwhile and probably are. But become involved in too many things and you'll find yourself skipping classes and assignments for meetings and activities.

Your success ultimately depends on how you do in those classes. Skip the meetings in favor of going to class. The best bet is to pick one organization that appeals to you and devote a predetermined amount of time to it every week. If you want to write for the school newspaper, figure out how much time you can spare, then talk to the editor. If your availability doesn't match the paper's needs, they may have to get along without you. If you want to be involved in the Young Republicans or Young Democrats, talk to the president of the organization. Find out what kinds of activities are planned to which you can contribute. But limit yourself, for the first term or two at least, to one organization.

A frightening number of students drop out of college, everywhere in the United States, during the first four weeks of every term. In some places, the number of students who finish the term is only half the number who began it. Don't become a statistic. Take a reasonable number of courses, work out a schedule with your adviser, take advantage of the various kinds of help available on campus, and sample a bit of college life. Above all, study. Remember your goals and work toward achieving them. Whatever they happen to be, explore your options. A little ingenuity in combining options, some patience, and a dollop of luck occasionally can achieve remarkable results. You'll soon realize that the college experience is one of the most enriching, rewarding experiences you could ever have.

CHAPTER FOUR

Heigh-Ho, Heigh-Ho: Entering the Job Market

W hen you think about finding a job, three questions should come into your mind:

- ◆ Do I have the training, or can I get the training, for it?
- ◆ Would I enjoy doing it?
- ◆ Do I really *want* to do it?

If you can answer yes to those three questions, there's nothing stopping you. We hope the last chapter gave you some suggestions and pointers that will help you answer the first question; we're going to try now to suggest some things you need to bear in mind when you answer the other two.

Note that we're going on the assumption that there's very little the disabled can't do. You should have the idea by now that we're convinced you can do whatever you want. Now you just have to do it. True, you might not wind up wheeling your way through musty, centuries-old Egyptian tombs, but it takes a special kind of person—disabled or not—to enjoy that kind of work anyway.

One of the most difficult aspects of the great job chase is deciding what you want to do. The possibilities seem limitless, and any number of options may present themselves. So how do you figure out what's right for you? A good way is to spend a few minutes thinking about what subjects in school interested you most. Then think about what subjects produced the best grades. If anything matches up, you almost certainly have aptitude in that area. But whether they're the same subjects or not, chances are you'll find a clue here to the kind of work you're best suited for. We've all known people, certainly, who seem to have "fallen into" the perfect profession. But those people are as few and far between as lottery winners. More realistically, when you ask people how they selected their chosen professions they'll tell you some kind of story related to school and the courses they took in some way.

When you consider job possibilities also remember that, whether you plan to work for someone or you're contemplating a home-based business, you're committing about one-third of your life to this activity. You'd better look at it from all sides and make sure it's something that will hold your interest and attention for a period of time. As you build a job history (that is, as you move up the professional ladder) you'll be viewed as something of a grass-hopper if you display a tendency to change jobs every year or so. Likewise, if you have your own business, but change what you do from time to time, you might find you have the reputation of someone who can't "sit still" in a business. We're not saying that you need to pick something, then stagnate in it. Far from it. We're suggesting that you commit yourself to developing your skills within an area, then seek your variations within that area, too.

This chapter is divided into two parts. The first part deals with job-hunting when you want to get outside your home to work; the second concerns starting your own business at home. The information presented in both parts and by a variety of people is

Employment Publications

Several publications that deal with employment and the disabled:

Exploring Computer Careers for the Handicapped by Marilyn Jones, 1985, $8.95, The Rosen Publishing Group, Inc., 29 East 21st St., New York, N.Y. 10010; (212) 777-3017.

This 149-page book offers information on training programs such as those of the Association of Rehabilitation Programs in Data Processing and home-based programs. Specific peripherals are presented and their uses are described for a variety of disability groups. Jones refers to numerous disabled consumers computers and those involved in training, continuing education, and the development of computer aids and devices. Other topics are aptitude testing and evaluation, independent living and interviewing, cottage industries and computer repair, engineering, and education. Each program is described, with the address included.

Health and Job Retention: The Arbitrator's Perspective by Terry Leap, 1984, $6.00, ILR Press, New York State School of Industrial and Labor Relations, Cornell University, Ithaca, N.Y. 14853; (607) 256-2264.

This 54-page publication for personnel administrators, supervisors, health professionals, and others concerned with labor and management relations discusses 144 arbitration decisions concerning the grievances related to the employment rights of employees with chronic or age-related health problems. The analysis of these cases provides information on the legal responsibilities of employers and

tried and true. But it can only work for you if you let it. Take it in the spirit with which it is intended—as guidance—and it can lead you to a rewarding career.

Job hunting

We've all heard people who bemoan the fact that they can't find a job. Chances are, one reason is that they've taken a scattershot unions as well as the standards and criteria often used by arbitrators in reaching their decisions.

Disabled Persons in the Workplace: An Introductory Reference and Resource Guide, edited by Lee Magnolia and Donna Mandelstam. Free from Electronic Industries Foundation, Project with Industry, 2001 Eye St., N.W., Washington, D.C. 20006.

Includes an annotated bibliography of publications on accommodation aids, attitudes, devices, employment equipment, evaluation, and services related to disabled persons, along with a listing of organizations that offer a variety of services to disabled persons and their employers.

Jobs for Disabled People by Frank Bowe, $1.00, Public Affairs Pamphlets, 381 Park Ave. S., New York, N.Y. 10016.

Addresses patterns of employment and income, rights and responsibilities, accommodation aids and devices, special programs that help and new challenges for persons who have disabilities. It also lists a number of helpful resources.

Technology and Rehabilitation of Disabled Persons in the Information Age, edited by Leonard Perlmen, $10.00, NRA, 633 S. Washington St., Alexandria, Va. 22314.

The report of the eighth Mary E. Switzer Memorial Seminar. Key issues such as employment and training opportunities and the impact of high technology on the rehabilitation professional are covered.

Disabled Women in America: A Statistical Report Drawn from U.S. Census Data by Frank Bowe, 1984. Free from The President's Committee on Employment of the Handicapped, Washington, D.C. 20210.

Reports on the working status of disabled women in the United States. Among the statistics are income and rates of employment.

approach—they've randomly called on and applied at a variety of places with little rhyme or reason, and even less organization.

Job hunting is certainly not a science any of us wants to practice for an extended period; rather, we'd prefer to be successful the first time out and land the job that will help us live happily ever after. We may or may not have that happen, but we can improve our chances by approaching the project methodically.

First, develop a list of a dozen or so prospective employers. Find out if they're hiring in the area that fits your skills. A simple call to the personnel department of most companies will tell you that. All you have to ask is "Are you taking applications for ———— ?" If the answer is positive, get an application in as soon as possible. If it's negative, ask if there's a target date when the organization will be accepting applications. You can save yourself a lot of grief and energy that way.

Another often-overlooked way to find out who's in the market for people with your training is to check at the placement office at your local college. If you got your degree there, so much the better, but don't let that keep you away. Most job placement offices maintain a bulletin board for job announcements in an easily accessible location. Take a notebook with you when you go so that you can write down information. You'll probably come away with a list of leads. One other tip: job placement bulletin boards are continually being updated; check every week or so if you possibly can.

Be sure to consider employment possibilities in municipal, county, state, or federal government. For one thing, with government offices you never need to be concerned about your disability being an issue. Remember: the government wrote the laws concerning equal access and opportunity for the disabled. All government offices will certainly meet all government standards on that score, even if they may be shorthanded or underbudgeted.

To find out about government job possibilities in your area, merely look up the personnel office for each type (municipal, county, state, or federal) in the phone book. Some phone books even list the government agencies in a separate section, making the job that much easier for you. Just call and ask where job announcements are posted. In some regions, you can even be put on a mailing list to receive job announcements for a period of time. You may find that not every job in government comes through this central office, but many do. Keep an eye on magazines for the disabled, too—*Accent, Mainstream, Together,* and others (they're listed in the appendix). They often carry ads for government jobs.

Suppose, though, that you have a degree in education or in business administration and want to teach. Or that you're a computer whiz anxious to help some agency get organized and start saving taxpayer dollars. What then? Isn't that when you want to burst right into the president's office and announce your presence? Absolutely not! Instead, for more specialized jobs in government, you need to spend a bit more time on the phone. Call various organizations' personnel offices and ask if they have positions (*not* whether they're hiring; just whether they have positions) in your particular skill area. Build a list that way.

Most agencies will send you an application by mail. It's a good idea to go ahead and fill it out. Normally, applications are kept on file for a year. In a perfect world, if a job opening comes up and you're qualified, you'll automatically be considered. It's not a bad idea, though, to visit those agencies from time to time and check the personnel board. When an opening does come up and you're interested, ask the personnel people to make sure your application is included in that job's pool.

Not every job search will be handled the same way. For some, you might need to take an aptitude test. For others, you may be able to learn of openings by going to a specific office. Learn to pick up the phone and call with your questions. Generally, you'll get directed the right way, even though you may have to ask for clarification. The important thing is not to be afraid to ask.

Have a top-notch résumé

At the same time you're developing your list of employers, be sure you keep your résumé (or whatever you choose to call it) up to date. Numerous businesses will prepare your résumé for a fee, of course, but you might just as easily do it yourself.

Remember three things about a résumé: keep it current, keep it specific to the kinds of job you're applying for, and keep it simple. Most employers will tell you a résumé should be updated every year, more often if significant changes occur. We suggest every six months as a matter of routine. You never know when something might come up, and you'll want to have your résumé ready.

Many experts suggest that your résumé should be organized differently for different types of jobs and even different types of application procedures. According to this advice, then, someone with public relations experience who's interested in becoming a teacher might do the résumé one way when applying for teaching jobs and another when applying for public relations positions. However, if the school wants a teacher with professional experience, the résumé would be prepared to emphasize employment in public relations, and—well, you get the idea. It can be confusing, yes, but it can no doubt be productive. For most of us, though, one résumé will suffice.

Keeping a résumé simple can be hard to do. Our tendency, especially as we enjoy some success in our field, is to cram the résumé full of every detail imaginable. Fight that tendency. Organize it by education (high school and college only), professional experience in the field, related professional experience (if applicable), honors and awards you've received, professional organizations, and personal information. Some chief executive officers have said that a résumé longer than two pages is too long. Others establish three pages as a limit. If that's what CEOs think, it ought to influence how you prepare your résumé.

A few years ago, résumés on colored paper were all the rage. The idea was that a different color would stand out from the normal white. Eventually, of course, most applicants were using paper of different colors, and it was the normal *white* which stood out. But, remember, it's what's *on* the page that counts, not what color the page is. Still, we recommend basic white as the best choice for a simple and professional-looking résumé.

You might wonder at all this concentration on the résumé. The reason is simple: the résumé is your foot in the door for any job. In most cases, the people screening applications haven't seen you, and only rarely will they know who you are at all. So your résumé has to catch an eye and "sell" the screeners on the idea of talking to you.

You say you don't have enough to put on a résumé to make it impressive? Think again. One homemaker in Colorado who found herself forty and displaced, who had never worked outside the home before, prepared a résumé based on her homemaking duties. She identified herself as a qualified budget manager, dietitian, bookkeeper, teacher, domestic, cook, recreation director, nurse, fashion consultant, and psychologist. The first CEO who saw this woman's résumé hired her. Her creativity and analytic ability impressed him. The woman had attended a résumé-writing workshop at a local community college and had gotten the idea there. Such workshops, usually one-day affairs, are offered regularly and offer tips on what's current. Consider taking one of these, especially if you're writing your first résumé.

The interview: What will I say?

You've submitted a first-class résumé and it's caught the eye of the personnel director. You've received a call inviting you to an interview (this might be an appropriate point to mention your disability, by the way). The day has come, your big moment has arrived, and you're scared to death you won't be able to say a word once you get in there.

We could tell you to relax until tomorrow, and it wouldn't help. Perhaps this will: your résumé has already done 90 percent of the work. You've been invited in because these people have already identified you as one of three or four people *they* would like to have on board. You're a winner going in, and you're being interviewed for just a few reasons: they want to meet you, they want to make sure you're articulate, and they want to make sure you aren't one of those rare people (oh, yes, they're out there) who look great on paper but don't measure up in person. Since you already know you've got items two and three covered, the only reason left to go in there is because your new boss wants to meet you. So relax. You'll do fine. (It's true, you know: the more relaxed you are, the better you'll do.)

Before you go to the interview, though, you should run through a few quick things. First, make sure your clothes are appropriate. It would hardly do, for instance, to interview for a job as a banker while dressed in sweatshirt and jeans.

As for the interview itself, read over the advice elsewhere in this chapter. Take it to heart. Answer questions frankly and, above all, pleasantly. Keep a smile on your face. Near the end of the interview you'll usually get a chance to ask a question or two. If you aren't familiar with it, you might inquire about accessibility to the building, the work area, restrooms, lounges, and whatever else. Ask in a straightforward manner; don't be belligerent or confrontational. You might, for instance, ask how long it might

Clothing—A Silent Communicator
BY GERALDINE RAY

Research indicates appearance is a major source of information during a job interview. Dress is a prominent factor of appearance. Individuals (regardless of physical limitations) are judged on the basis of their appearance before verbal interactions take place. Clothing is considered an acceptable, as well as a significant, means of nonverbal communication. To realize social and business success, the "right" clothing is imperative.

A research project [in 1987] was conducted to determine if dress would affect the ratings made on personal characteristics of physically impaired individuals. Ninety-four managers were asked to read a job description and then rate three men in wheelchairs. Each of the three wore a different level of dress—high, moderate or low. The levels of dress were constructed from business attire recommendations of John T. Molloy in *Dress for Success* (1975). The job applicant at the high appropriateness-of-dress level wore a dark gray pinstripe suit with vest; white, long-sleeved shirt; and maroon polka-dot tie. The model dressed in moderately appropriate clothing wore a light blue sports coat, dark blue pants, white shirt, and dark-blue and light-blue striped tie. For low appropriateness of dress the model was clad in a hot-pink and dark-blue plaid sports coat, dark blue pants, gray shirt, and no tie.

Findings seem conclusive—dress definitely affected ratings. The better the dress of the physically impaired job applicant, the higher the ratings in other areas such as competence and motivation.

The ninety-four managers were also asked their willingness to hire the job applicants based on their dress. Dress had a highly significant effect on the decision to hire an applicant. The more appropriate the dress, the more likely the person was to recommend hiring the job applicant. Several respondents indicated that the job applicant wearing the low level of dress should wear a necktie.

take for a ramp for your wheelchair to be installed, rather than saying, "You understand that the law requires that you install a ramp." You might also inquire into health and retirement benefits. Such a question often signals to an employer that you're expecting to spend a career with an organization. Avoid asking about vacations and holidays—you're applying for a *job*, not for a paid vacation.

The New York Times reported in 1989 that the labor pool in America is shrinking because of retirements and other factors. As a result, doors are opening for jobs for millions of disabled workers who hadn't been able to find work to this point. The decade ahead will be one of expanding opportunities for the disabled. Plan to take advantage of those opportunities.

Working at home

One work option you should be aware of, if you aren't already, for the coming decade is the increased opportunity for working at home. In major cities this alternative is becoming more and more a reality, and it requires only that the employee have an area in the house or apartment to which he/she can go and find relative quiet every day. The company installs a computer workstation and connects it by phone line to the central office. The employee may go into the office once or twice a week to deliver or pick up materials, but generally he or she receives work via the company's electronic mail system, completes it, and transmits it back to the main office.

Any number of jobs exist that can be done from home today, thanks to computers. A brief listing might include abstracter, budget analyst, columnist, city manager, desktop publisher, insurance claims representative, lawyer, reservations agent, researcher— well, you get the idea.

For an employer, the advantages are numerous: increased productivity by you, reduced space needs (which can mean lower rent), lower overhead, and employee retraining possibilities, among other things. For you, the advantages are obvious: no traffic to fight, tremendous flexibility, no dress restrictions, no worktime limitations. Beware, however; some of these advantages can become disadvantages. Such easy access means a stronger tendency to workaholism. It also means you forgo the companionship of fellow workers.

Your Job Interview: How to Answer the Unasked Questions
BY M. HOPKINS-BEST

Getting through a job interview is one of the major hurdles to getting a job. Many employers must comply with affirmative action policies which require hiring people with disabilities. However, anyone would rather be hired for his qualifications, rather than as the "token" disabled employee. Therefore, it is critical to present a positive, capable image during the job interview. Most employers have concerns or questions about the disability they may not ask in the interview. This is the "hidden agenda" of a job interview. You should respond to these concerns even if they are not raised. Typical hidden questions and suggestions for addressing them are:

Will you miss a lot of work because of your disability?

Whether or not an employer asks about your ability to attend work regularly, find opportunities to stress your good attendance at other jobs, rehabilitation programs, school, or whatever you can. If you know you will need to miss work for surgery or some other anticipated event, tell the employer and emphasize that you would want to arrange compensatory time. If you need to work a flextime schedule, be straightforward about your job needs. Avoid referring to your disability as "illness" or "sickness." Emphasize your interest in good nutrition and physical fitness activities which enhance your good health.

Will you really be able to do the work?

Individuals who are "fresh" out of a training program are particularly vulnerable to this concern. Training program requirements may not have been comparable to job requirements; for example, you may have been sitting in a classroom to learn a physically demanding job. Bring up successful educational field experiences, volunteer activities, or paid work that required task performance similar to the job. Answer questions honestly about the effect of your disability on your ability to perform any job tasks, but be ready to suggest ways of making accommodations if needed. Don't leave it up to the employer to guess whether you can do the work with or without accommodations—he may underestimate you! If you have had previous jobs, discuss tasks you performed successfully that apply to the desired job, even if the job titles are dissimilar.

Will the other employees accept you?

While you should not have to relieve others' anxieties about differences, remember that the employer has a vested interest in the psychological comfort of his current employees. As unfair as it may be, you have to appear willing to make an assertive effort to "fit in." Talk about your social and professional interactions with other people. For example, tell how you enjoyed taking part in the Newcomer's Club so you could get to know people in your community. Discuss any experiences you have had in a leadership role. Make sure the social activities you describe are not limited to interactions only with other disabled people. Don't overlook the importance of creating a favorable impression with the receptionist before your interview. Many employers ask their receptionists for an informal assessment of how applicants acted before putting on their "interview face."

What do I have to do to accommodate your disability?

Most employers do not have expertise in job accommodations but may be embarrassed about their lack of knowledge. You should suggest any necessary modifications for the job. Do your homework before the job interview so you will have a clear understanding of the job tasks. Emphasize your abilities and independence. For example, if you are visually impaired, tell how easy it was to locate the employer's office because the building is well organized. Respond to questions such as "Who dresses you?" with humor and grace. Try not to be defensive; remember most able-bodied people are educable.

Is your training legitimate?

Some employers will wonder if you were "passed through" your education because of your disability. Emphasize the requirements of your educational program(s), the competitiveness of your field of training, and how you enjoyed the challenge of a rigorous training program. If modifications were made in educational experience and/or previous jobs, emphasize that standards were not reduced (for example, tests taken orally required the same level of performance).

If the employer asks these questions, give him credit for honesty. However, if the interviewer does not ask any of these questions overtly, you should respond to these concerns while answering other questions. When asked for additional information or an open-ended statement is made, such as "tell me about yourself," provide excellent opportunities to present a capable image. If these concerns are addressed, the employer will have a more thorough understanding of your real abilities.

The Job Accommodation Network

Since 1984 the federal government has operated the Job Accommodation Network, a computer system designed to help potential employers of the disabled. By doing so the government hopes that more employers will hire disabled workers. JAN offers employers advice for adapting workstations to accommodate the disabled. When employers call they get names and numbers of other employers who have dealt with accommodation problems. They also receive information about devices that help accommodate the disabled.

JAN was created by the President's Committee on Employment of the Handicapped. It can be reached at 1-800-526-7234 (1-800-JAN-PCEH).

Insurance companies, especially, have already enjoyed success with this work-at-home system. Estimates have been published that, by the turn of the century, 60 percent of the office workers in central London, England, will work at home—simply because of the cost of office space. Work-at-home schemes save the company money on building rent, and they save employees the hassle of fighting urban traffic jams twice every day. For the disabled worker, the possibility of working at home appears likely to open even more doors for jobs in the years ahead.

Running your own business

Perhaps the idea of operating your own business from your home appeals to you. Or perhaps you can or want to do something but can't get out of the house. Either way, making a success of something you run yourself is particularly satisfying because of what it says about your self-sufficiency.

Businesses run from the home can produce tidy incomes but they require constant attention. Let's suppose you need to close down your operation next month because you have to have some medical work done and you'll be away from home for four days. You need to notify your regular customers and suppliers now, so they can plan for their needs while you're gone. Advance planning is one of the most important aspects of running a home business.

It's often been said that Americans have a remarkable way of identifying a need, then finding a way to fill that need. When you set up a business, you should consider certain things before you open your doors, however:

- Whether your disability will hamper your ability to care for your inventory (stock your shelves, etc.)
- Whether you can physically handle the many aspects of running a business
- If you're dealing with raw materials, whether they might have any impact on your disability (talk to your doctor)
- Whether your business could stand to be closed for a prolonged period if you need surgery or are otherwise laid up for some time.

For an able-bodied person, let alone someone who's disabled, the hassles of starting up and running a business can be exasperating. You need to make certain you keep a watchful eye on your health as you scurry around finding suppliers and lining up wholesalers. You won't do yourself any good if you have to postpone your grand opening because you're in the hospital after running yourself ragged.

No matter what city or state you live in, you'll have to wind your way through a maze of licenses and permits to start a business in your home. An attorney, if you can afford one, can help make this less stressful. If you can't, you'll need to spend some time on the phone and visiting offices yourself. First, call the city planning commission. Identify yourself as a disabled person starting a home business, since some states have less restrictive laws for the disabled. If you expect customers to be coming to your home in large numbers you may need to apply for what's called a zoning variance, if you live in an area the city has determined should be free of businesses. The person you talk to will ask a specific series of questions about your proposed business and will tell you if you need a variance. If you do, ask to have the necessary documents sent to you.

You'll also have to get business licenses, usually from the city and state, and set up a sales tax account with the state (which is done by simply writing to your state's revenue department for the

---

A Success Story

Helynn's friend Lillian, who was born with a small, underdeveloped leg and uses crutches, turned the front room of her family's Victorian house into an inviting, colorful, and cozy needlework shop where neighbors from miles around gravitated when they wanted a chat and a skein of yarn for a sweater. Lillian used floor-to-ceiling bookshelves to display knitting yarn and silk embroidery floss. A coffee table held books of instruction, and comfortable chairs invited her guests/customers to sit and relax.

The bright, friendly atmosphere in the place kept the customers coming back. Lillian also knew her business and offered the newest yarns and patterns; there was nothing stuffy or old-fashioned about her shop. She also knew how to knit, cross-stitch, and do needlepoint, and she cheerfully instructed beginners.

It doesn't really take a special sort of person to make a go of this kind of business, as long as you enjoy what you're doing. With a little creativity you can turn your home into a rewarding business, with very little cash outlay at the start.

---

appropriate form), and you'll want to insure your inventory or increase your liability insurance. Your insurance agent can help with the latter, but at this point, too, you'll want to secure the services of a good tax adviser for help with many other details. Always identify yourself as disabled, because you may qualify for incentives or other benefits.

So far, we've generally assumed that you'll be turning your home into a storefront and that customers will be parking their cars all over the neighborhood. That may not be the case. You can run plenty of businesses that provide services rather than goods; if that's the case, the paperwork will be easier. One disabled woman ran a booking service for limousines. Virtually all of her business was conducted by phone. A disabled man did tax work for a number of small businesses that were equipped with computers and modems. He saw his clients only occasionally; the rest of the time they transmitted all the information he needed by computer.

Make sure that you have a specific area of your home set up for conducting business. The Internal Revenue Service requires, for an office-in-home deduction, a room that is used *exclusively* for the kind of work you do. Let's say, then, that you sell trophies and other such award gadgetry (a business with a high markup, by the way). To meet IRS guidelines, you'd have to use one room exclusively for a showroom and for conducting business—taking orders, storing shipments, and deliveries. Normally, it isn't hard to find some part of the house to partition off; it's just important to be aware of the requirement. Your tax adviser can help you with other requirements that will save you money.

We don't mean to scare you away from starting your own business by detailing all the things you have to do. Yes, it does take somewhat more work to start a business than to go to work for someone else. But the rewards can be greater, too. And we don't mean those intangible rewards of good feelings about self-sufficiency and contributing to the free enterprise system, although those things almost certainly enter into our thinking from time to time. No, there are more tangible benefits, and your tax adviser will help you identify most of them. One is that you, as an individual, won't have to pay any income taxes, or a very limited amount. Instead of taking a salary from your company, your tax adviser will show you how to set up and take what are called "owner's draws." Income tax liability on these is significantly different from salaries. We aren't tax consultants, certainly, and so we encourage you to talk to your tax adviser for other benefits that accrue from operating your own business. They can be considerable.

Obviously, one thing you'll need to do is figure out how to get customers once you're in business. You can rely on word of mouth—which carries a remarkable degree of reliability, especially when an operation is extremely good or extremely bad. Certainly, your friends and acquaintances will talk about your business, and you'll probably generate some income that way. But don't overlook advertising. Often, for in-home businesses, a small ad in the Yellow Pages can be your biggest benefactor. Such ads usually aren't cheap, but the cost is billed out on a monthly basis (with your phone bill). But when people are looking for, say, a desktop

SBA Aid

The federal Small Business Administration operates several different programs, including at least one special small business loan program for the disabled.

A call to the SBA's contact person for the Handicapped Assistance Loan (HAL) will get you all the information and material you can absorb. But the SBA may have other programs that can help you. Tell the person you talk to what you're setting out to do and ask what special assistance programs are available besides HAL that might be applicable to you.

Try a nearby SBA office, if you have one in your area, but for the most recent information about the HAL program, you might be better off calling the Washington office:

Small Business Administration
1441 L St., N.W., Room 418
Washington, D.C. 20416
(202) 653-6765 (Voice/TDD)

Here are two toll-free numbers which might help you with specific questions about starting and financing a small business:

The Small Business Administration Answer Desk, 1-800-368-5855, offers advice to business owners and potential owners about starting a business, financing it, overcoming problems, and contracting with the government.

The Small Business Advisory Service Hotline, 1-800-424-5201, has information about import/export programs and works specifically with ways to facilitate export financing.

publishing service, the first place they usually look is the Yellow Pages. Call and ask to meet with a sales representative. **Tip:** If you're going to spend the money to advertise in the Yellow Pages, spend a bit extra and get a small display ad. It will generate more calls than a line listing.

Cash limitations can seem a significant deterrent when starting a home business. But several avenues are open to you. The federal government, through the Small Business Administration, offers low-interest loans to help start small businesses. Some states do also. For information on these programs, call the phone numbers listed elsewhere in this chapter. If for some reason you'd prefer not to deal with the government, don't be afraid to see your local banker about a start-up loan. But before you do, prepare a year's worth of projections about how you expect the business's finances to progress. That way you'll be able to show that you've thought seriously about your business's future.

Go back now and reread the sections on interviewing for a job and dressing for work. The same things apply when you operate your own business. View yourself as a business professional who operates a business every day of the week. Dress like a professional and operate your business during regular hours. Have business cards printed. Join the local Chamber of Commerce, if you can, and try to attend their activities. You'll meet other businesspeople this way and, in time, you'll expand your network of contacts. Give out business cards freely. Leave your cards in places where they might be picked up by interested people. In short, work at generating business. And one final bit of advice: attend a small business seminar at least once a year to keep yourself up to date.

A number of excellent books on the market can help you explore every aspect of setting up a home-based business. Pick up one or two. They'll give you ideas about possibilities you hadn't thought of and they'll cover virtually every detail involved in getting your business going and keeping it going.

Here are just a few of the businesses disabled people—even the severely disabled—have successfully run from their homes: secretarial services, bookkeeper (churches, especially, are good potential clients, and a bookkeeping service can be established for little expense), artist, poet (although, sadly, poetry doesn't pay anyone much money these days), commercial printer (really!), desktop publisher (thanks to computers), booking agency for nightclubs, seamstress and/or tailor, and dealer in various collectibles. This is far from an exhaustive list. The books we mentioned above will be far more exhaustive. This list is just to whet your appetite and to demonstrate that you *can* operate a successful business from home. You're only limited by your imagination and willingness to work.

CHAPTER FIVE

Gadgets Galore

From plastic saucers you can throw around to electronic devices that help cerebral palsy victims walk, gadgets are everywhere. Enterprising people have devoted untold hours and countless dollars designing ingenious creations to make our lives easier and more comfortable. We live in a gadget-oriented world, and the advent of the age of technology has only heightened that preoccupation with gadgets.

Nowhere is the concentration of gadgetry more evident than in aids for the disabled. The market is an obvious one, and a flood of companies—small to gigantic—has filled people's needs with a seemingly endless array of devices and trinkets, from implanted electrodes to control muscle spasms to dishes with a barrier so food doesn't slide off onto the table. It's like that neighbor whose garage was filled with tools—the one who always said that if he didn't have it, you probably didn't need it.

This chapter does not attempt to identify or discuss all the things available to assist the disabled. But we hope it will give you a look at the gadgetry you can adapt to your specific needs— whether a computer to help you work, a device to increase comfort or enhance communication and mobility, software to help you learn, or something to make life easier and more convenient—and that the list of companies and organizations in the appendix can help you track down the specific device you need. If you know where to look, you can find almost anything a disabled person could possibly want or need.

Gadgetry has taken a different direction recently, and the newest generation of such devices is perhaps more efficient and more beneficial for the disabled than ever before. The invention of the microchip has pushed technology into areas never thought possible and, thankfully, pushed prices down. These days, with few exceptions, most things you could want are affordable. And, by starting with a basic computer system and expanding from there, the sky is virtually the only limit to disabled access.

That such gadgetry is beneficial is unquestionable. However, as David Young in Denver cautions in an article in *Science & Technology for the Handicapped*, many so-called special needs devices can be equaled or surpassed, both in price and usefulness, by products available to the general public. This doesn't mean that you should avoid specially designed aids for the disabled. It merely reminds all of us, disabled or not, to shop around before we spend our money.

Still, the coming of the computer age has meant the availability of countless new devices and tools specifically designed to help the disabled. These creations, sometimes called peripheral devices as well as computer software, have helped open a whole new world to the disabled.

Enter the computer world

First, you have to have a computer. Why? Many have said that computers help the disabled live closer to the mainstream of society today than ever before. Francisco Villarruel, at the Trace Center on Computer Access for Handicapped Individuals at the University of Wisconsin/Madison, told the Associated Press in June 1984 that approximately two and a half million disabled people who had once been incapable of work could now communicate and work because of computer innovations. The number has increased even more since then, thanks to computer technology.

Dr. Lawrence Scadden of the Electronic Industries Association, a Washington, D.C.-based trade organization, told *The New York Times* in June 1988 that "the microcomputer has been the most valuable piece of technology ever developed to assist disabled people." You've already seen (in Chapter 3) how a computer can connect you to a college classroom from your living room or bedroom and enable you to earn a college degree without leaving your home. A computer can also help you run a business from your home. It can keep an up-to-date inventory and store records for your business; it can create and print invoices; it can even help you make tough business decisions. A dozen years ago, the effort required for a disabled person to operate a business was great and the opportunities limited. Today, thanks to computers, the effort is minimal and the opportunities great. Disabled people across the country now run everything from catering and secretarial services to limousine rental and mail order shopping agencies—all with the help of a computer. If you need further convincing, remember that renowned astrophysicist Stephen Hawking could not have written his best-selling *A Brief History of Time* without a computer: he can no longer speak and can only communicate through a computer.

If you're like many people, you're a bit intimidated by the technology—or at least by the terminology. Don't worry. Everybody feels that way about something new. Look at it this way: a computer is only a tool. It is mindless. It can only do what you tell it to do. And, short of dropping it on the floor, you can't break it easily. If these thoughts don't ease your concerns, consider taking a computer-literacy course at your local community college. Or, at the very least, do a little reading on computer basics.

Computers perform mundane tasks routinely, freeing our minds for other things. Computers can balance a checkbook, figure income tax, store business records, calculate loan payments, keep phone lists, address envelopes, send and receive Morse code, play games, help you learn to type, make writing easier, check your spelling and grammar, keep lists of things to do, display actual photographs, do research, and enable you to communicate with people and other computers around the world (depending on the size of your telephone budget, of course). The possibilities, more than ever before, are endless.

Selecting your new friend

This book has said again and again that computers are going to play an ever-increasing role in American life, and that bears repeating here. Few of us really doubt that computers can perform a great many valuable tasks. But many of us aren't sure we have any use for those applications in day-to-day living, because we aren't sure exactly what computers do and how to make them work for us. Computers are really simple devices (for the "end user"—us). In fact, for many who are disabled—those able to use the keyboard—a basic computer system is all that's necessary. But technological devices for the disabled have gone far beyond that, and an impressive range of special devices are available today. Before we look at specifically disabled-oriented devices, let's examine just what goes into a basic computer system.

The most basic computer systems can be had for as little as $400, although the cost goes up significantly from there. Do yourself a favor from the start, though, and don't skimp. If you don't add a few important extras at the beginning, you either soon will or you'll give up on the machine and wind up owning an expensive doorstop. You'll spend more money all at once, certainly, but with the proper setup you'll soon wonder how you ever got along without it.

The first consideration in a computer is its "brain" or central processing unit. Stick with the major operating systems—IBM (sometimes called PC-DOS or MS-DOS; the "DOS" stands for Disk Operating System, which runs the programs) or Apple. Those two pioneered the home computer industry, have made the greatest advances, and will be around for a long time to come. They have set the standard for the computer industry and, as a result, for computer-compatibile devices for the disabled. Various companies produce knockoffs or clones of IBM systems, and many are excellent buys. Others may not be as good. To get an idea, pick up a copy of *Computer Buyer's Guide*, an annual publication, at your local newsstand, or read a few copies of one of the many magazines for IBM and Apple users. Talk to friends who use computers and to members of user's groups (clubs of computer owners; any computer sales clerk should be able to give you at least one name). Be sure the operating system is standard; that makes repairs or replacement parts easier to take care of and cheaper in the long run.

The next consideration is the display. On a limited budget, a monochrome (single-color) display will work fine. But a color monitor, which costs a couple of hundred dollars more (with the necessary interface, or circuitry, that sends the proper signals from the computer to the monitor), is easier on the eyes. Monochrome monitors usually come in amber, green, or white. Test all three if that's the display you're committed to, to see which will result in the least eyestrain. A color display (usually called CGA, for color graphics adapter) allows you to change colors whenever you want. If you plan to spend many hours a day working at the computer, you might consider the extra expense (another $300 to $500) of an EGA (enhanced graphics adapter) or VGA (video graphics adapter) color monitor. Those displays generate extremely high resolution. Suppose you're writing a book or entering large amounts of numbers and you're working with green characters on a black background; it's just a matter of a keystroke or two to change to yellow characters on a blue background if your eyes get tired. And the resolution is clear: you won't have trouble distinguishing one character from another.

The next integral part of the basic computer system is the disk drive. The cheapest computer packages (the ones you see advertised in the newspaper every week) come with one floppy disk drive. A second floppy drive or a hard drive costs extra, but it's money well spent. Floppy disks are small, flimsy things encased in heavy paper, cardboard, or plastic on which the computer magnetically records the data you produce. One of these small wonders can hold about the equivalent of 45,000 words, or roughly 165 typewritten pages, double-spaced. In other words, one disk can store a short novel. The programs necessary to make your computer do things come on floppy disks. They're about the size of a compact disk—five and a quarter inches in diameter (they come in three-and-a-half-inch diameter, too)—and they have to be inserted into and removed from the disk drive, the device that operates roughly like a record player and "reads" the information from the disk into the computer's memory. Many of the most efficient and convenient pieces of software cease to be efficient or convenient if you have only one disk drive, however. A full-featured word processor, for example, will require one program disk, one data disk (to store the information you've written), one disk for the dictionary to check your spelling, another for the thesaurus (to help you find the right word more easily), and another with the necessary information to link your printer to your computer. You can see already that, to do serious word processing, a single-drive system could have you spending more time changing disks than working.

A dual-drive system is obviously better and costs about $80 to $100 more. But the real answer, especially for the disabled, is what's called a hard or fixed disk. This kind of disk costs between $225 and $700 (including the interface device to make it work with your computer), depending on the storage capacity of the disk. The smallest hard disks now available hold 20 megabytes of information—the equivalent of about 60 floppy disks (or 9,900 typewritten, double-spaced pages). Already you can see the advantage of a hard drive: the programs you need or want to have handy, and the information you've stored, are all in one place and already installed when you turn the computer on. No need to search for the right disk or to put a disk in the drive.

A typical hard drive will store the main programs you'll use most: a word processor, a spreadsheet for bookkeeping or other purposes, a filing system, a program to enable telephone communication with other computers, perhaps a few games and other diversion-type programs, the data you've saved, and the computer operating system. The only limitation to what you can put on a hard drive is the capacity of the drive itself and the size of your pocketbook.

Software makes it all go

After the basic computer system—central processing unit, monitor, keyboard (which comes with the system), and drive system—the next thing to consider is software. Naturally, you'll want to take home some software to use with your new computer. Your dealer will probably provide you with the most recent version of the Disk Operating System for your computer type and perhaps a disk or two of public domain games or other programs. If you want to add to that right away, choose a relatively inexpensive commercial program with a number of applications. A program like PFS: Professional File, for example, is an electronic filing cabinet that allows you to design forms any way you want and provides quick data retrieval. It's also extremely simple to learn, has all commands at the bottom of the screen all the time, and has on-screen help available every step of the way. You can use one "file" as an address book, another for business data, another for ideas, another for bibliographies for term papers, and another for mailing labels (it will format and print those, too). You may not use it forever, but it's versatile enough that you won't be wasting money if you buy it now and add more specific software later.

The key to buying commercial software is to test it before you buy. Read whatever you can find about it. Check with others who may have used it. Try it out if you can. Once you've bought it, don't be afraid to experiment. Software manufacturers tell you to make a copy of the master disk or disks immediately. Then if you crash (destroy) the program, you can always dig out the master disk and start again. All you'll have lost is a little time. Finally, when you do buy software, keep the manufacturer's phone number handy. Most software companies maintain an 800 number for what they call "customer support." The people they employ are hired specifically to answer your questions. Call them if you can't find the answer in the instruction manual.

You can cut through the software jungle by knowing before you go shopping precisely what you want to do with a computer. If you plan to spend most of your time writing, then a word processor should probably be your primary purchase. For record-keeping for your business at home, consider one of the many spreadsheet programs.

A variety of more detailed introductory computer books is available, and magazines can provide newcomers to computers with a great deal of useful information. Simply check your local bookstore and the magazine rack at most drug or grocery stores.

Putting it all together

When you set out to get a computer, get everything at once. If you don't, you'll soon want it anyway, and then you'll be without the machine for a period of time while the devices you buy later are installed. Some of the more basic add-ons you might consider include: a good printer, a graphics "card," a light pen or "mouse," and a modem.

The printer speaks for itself; thousands are on the market. They can be had for as little as $180 and as much as $4,000. The kind you choose should be determined by what you plan to do. If you expect to produce manuscripts, look for a printer which produces typewriter-quality pages (either a 24-pin dot matrix or a daisy wheel printer; the latter is slower but produces beautiful work). If you plan to produce newsletters or other typeset-quality work, a laser printer may be your answer—many college newspapers use them nowadays to produce all their pages. For printing reports, invoices, or statistics, one of the lower-priced dot matrix printers will no doubt do the job. No matter what you choose, however, make sure you see it in action and know it will do what you want before you buy it.

A graphics "card" is a circuit board that plugs into your machine and allows graphics (designs, photographs, and game-board layouts, among other things) to be displayed on your monitor. Most systems come with some sort of graphics card already installed, but you should check to make sure. Bought separately, the price can range from $80 to $400.

A light pen is simply a pen-shaped device that activates the computer with a beam of light. You select the item you want from a menu (the software is usually included) and touch the pen lightly

Carl and Karen Lambert

On a typical August Southern California morning in 1982, Karen Lambert's car overturned on the freeway on-ramp as she returned home from a flute lesson. She was thrown through the windshield and landed on the cement pavement, then run over by another car. Twelve hours of surgery to repair multiple fractures, a crushed shoulder and elbow, and a damaged liver followed. But she had also suffered a severe head injury. She lay in a coma eighty-one days and was not expected to live. Altogether she spent six months in the hospital, the first two in intensive care. When she came out of the coma, she was paralyzed on the left side and had severely diminished cognitive abilities, recalls her father, Carl.

Karen not only had to learn to walk again but also to swallow, talk, count, recognize the letters of the alphabet, and think. Karen received daily therapy in the hospital after she "awoke" from the coma. She went home with a wheelchair (from bed to wheelchair was, for her, a significant step forward) and returned to the hospital as an outpatient to continue therapy for another six months.

Carl, a retired naval officer and a computer expert, decided to stay home and devote his time to retraining Karen while Joyce, Karen's mother, continued her full-time job.

The monotony of repetitive training and the long hours involved can take their toll on therapist and patient alike. "To stimulate memory and concentration we played card games hour after hour," Carl remembers. "It was working slowly, but I had to come up with a different and easier approach. I finally began to wonder if a computer could be programmed to do my job and at the same time make it more fun for Karen."

Computers are good at repetitive tasks: they don't get bored, they don't get tired, and they don't complain. They unflaggingly perform the same task for as long as it takes for the patient-operator to learn it.

Carl, together with doctors, psychologists, and therapists (physical, occupational, and speech), worked out the problems involved in the multilevel retraining of a brain-damaged person. After developing a comprehensive view of what was involved, Carl began translating what he had learned into computer software. The programs he wrote had to help Karen learn by the same repetitive methods therapists and her father had used, and they had to be entertaining enough to keep her at the computer for several hours a day. They also had to increase in levels of difficulty as her ability to perform the prescribed routine improved.

Carl Lambert's computer program works mainly with cognitive abilities: concentration, memory, visual scanning, and speed of responses. "Without concentration you can't make decisions," he says. "Decisions require options. Options require memory." His programs offer entertaining (and therefore encouraging) feedback while they retrain the patient's cognitive abilities.

Karen was especially captivated by the poker game. In it, the computer deals out twenty-five cards at random and the player (the patient) selects the cards that will make the ten best poker hands. To do this, the brain must use its understanding of a concept as well as pattern recognition and problem solving. Simple games such as recognition of a letter of the alphabet are used in the beginning. From there the levels of difficulty are progressive.

Two years after the accident, Karen enrolled in algebra and French at Southwestern Community College in Chula Vista, California, and earned a B average. Today, she speaks clearly but slowly and walks with a slight limp. She has 80 percent use of her right hand, which had suffered extensive nerve damage.

Each year, about 200 people per 100,000 suffer severe head injuries. Of these, about 20 percent survive.

For the physically disabled or for brain-damaged individuals, staying alive is not enough. Those who survive need some degree of rehabilitation. Due in part to the rise in the accident rate and in part to the advances in medicine that make it possible for doctors to save lives, the number of patients and their families who can benefit from computer programs like Carl's increases each year.

"Ongoing guidance has to be part of the process," Carl points out. At the 300 hospitals and therapy centers around the nation that use the Lambert retraining process, the disabled and their families can get instruction and have continuous reinforcement as long as necessary.

The gains with this method of therapy are measured, first, in the patient's strides toward recovery; second, in the reduction of the tedious hours of retraining spent by the family; and third, in the significant reduction in the costs involved. Carl can be contacted about the software and the therapy centers at the address in the appendix.

Advances in software for computer-assisted retraining are being made constantly. To find out if similar software is available to help you, contact your local rehabilitation unit or the national office of the organization that deals with your disability.

against the screen. The computer goes to work. Such a device can be especially useful for the disabled, since the pressure required is minimal and the pen can be held in the mouth or attached to a pointer if necessary.

A mouse works in a somewhat similar way. It moves the cursor (the flashing line or box on the monitor screen that tells you where you are) around the screen as you move the small device around on a tabletop (like the light pen, it's connected to the computer by a cable). A mouse will have one to three buttons; you simply move the mouse until the cursor is where you want it, then press the proper button. Again, the computer goes to work. Both light pens and "mice" start at around $60. Either is very handy for anyone, disabled or not.

A modem links a computer and a telephone. It lets your computer communicate with other computers with similar setups. Like printers, modems come in a range of styles and prices. Two key things to remember about modems are an internal modem (installed *inside* your machine) means less to dust and less to clutter up your work area; avoid what are called "300 baud" modems. The term baud refers to the speed at which information can be transmitted over phone lines. The industry standard is 2,400 baud. A 300 baud modem, considered state-of-the-art a few years ago, is an antique today. It's simply too slow, and some systems won't accommodate it. A number of modems on the market cost only a few dollars and perform adequately. For the budget-minded, the mail-order discount houses advertise 1,200 baud internal modems every month for around $50. A 2,400 baud modem costs only about $25 more and doubles transmission speed.

Once you have a modem installed, an entire world of communications opens up to you and is as near as your keyboard. You can phone just about any other computer that is set up to receive calls. Most of these are called bulletin board systems. All you need is a phone number. You'll find an incredible variety of bulletin boards among the thousands around the country and overseas. Most are general-interest systems, but you'll soon learn that there are special-interest boards, too. They range in variety from dating services to medical information to centers where genealogists exchange information. Several are devoted specifically to information for the disabled, such as Alternative Inputs in Massachusetts, which is designed to address the special devices (computer and otherwise) needed by the disabled, and Montana Online, a resource center for both disabled people and senior citizens serving primarily Montana and surrounding states. Phone numbers of these and other similar bulletin boards appear in the appendix.

To develop your own starter list of phone numbers, pick up a copy of a publication called *Computer Shopper* (if you can't find it at your newsstand, you can write P.O. Box 1419, Titusville, Fla. 32781, for a copy). Every issue lists hundreds of electronic bulletin boards and identifies several by specialty. Most of those systems will give you a list of phone numbers for other systems you can call. Watch the long distance calls, though. It's easy to lose track of time when you're "on-line." On bulletin boards, you'll find an array of messages exchanged by callers on all sorts of topics. You'll soon find a thing or two you want to comment on. Before long, you'll be calling in for your electronic messages almost daily. In addition, you'll gain access to free software. Most bulletin boards maintain a wide selection of software, and you'll want to try some. You do that by downloading, or transferring electronically over the phone, the file from the master (host) computer to yours. The process is simple, and you're guided virtually every step of the way.

Nearly all bulletin boards are free (except for a possible long distance charge), but some have even attracted an international following. These charge a membership fee and are more complex to navigate than your favorite local system. They also charge by the hour, so you have to keep an eye on the clock when you call in. But they're usually worth the price. Three of the most popular, and most reasonable, for home computer users are CompuServe ($13.00 per hour for 1,200 baud), GEnie ($5 per hour), and Delphi ($7.20 per hour). Each carries more information than you could absorb in a lifetime. Each has up-to-the-minute news from several news wires, for instance, including Tass on some systems. Each offers a wide variety of forums, or special interest groups, where people can exchange ideas and questions.

Several major software manufacturers sponsor forums for their products—a handy place to take questions and pick up tips. You'll find a large collection of free software in each of these forums, too. You can also play games on-line, make travel arrangements, shop in an electronic "mall," and send private electronic mail to other users. You can even do research. Most maintain at least one electronic encyclopedia, but CompuServe can access more than 400 databases containing the full text of thousands of publications.

CompuServe also supports a forum devoted entirely to the disabled and disabilities. There the disabled individual can learn about new products coming on the market, read the most recent medical developments, and share questions and ideas with others on any subject—not just computers. But there's more: the software collection, most of which is contributed by members, contains hundreds of tips, tricks, addresses of organizations, and new ideas for dealing with disabilities. The forum is not restricted to any particular disability, either, and able-bodied members are welcome. CompuServe also carries the Handicapped Users' Database, an extensive and useful collection of up-to-date news, profiles, articles, and information about computer devices. For the disabled, these two forums alone are worth the price of the CompuServe membership.

These are not the only systems that offer such services. Dozens of others exist, but they are more expensive—some as much as $120 an hour plus a hefty membership fee. They're designed for businesspeople using those systems on company time. More detailed descriptions of several of them can be found in Alfred Glossbrenner's book *How to Look It up Online*.

Special devices for the disabled

Besides the fairly basic and commonly available computers and accompanying peripheral devices described here, an array of special equipment is available for Apple and IBM systems that has been designed specifically to help the disabled. One of the most common of these is the voice synthesizer—a gadget that "reads" printed or visual images (such as letters typed onto a computer monitor) and converts them into spoken words. Similar devices that translate standard characters into Braille are also widely available.

Depending on the disability and the need, devices exist that allow you to use the computer in a variety of ways: by direct contact with the keyboard or with the aid of a light pen, a head pointer, a mouthstick, or a handstick. You can push lightly on small buttons or large plates, sip and puff on a tube, or blink an eye. IBM and other companies even market a device called a "voice-activated keyboard utility" that allows control of computer programs using spoken commands. All the user has to do is "teach" the computer the commands and the voice; the computer will do the rest.

The Magic Wand keyboard is another example of the many kinds of keyboard enhancements available to assist the disabled. It can be operated from a sitting or reclining position and with limited one-hand movement or with a mouthstick. No force is required when touching the stylus (wand) to the keypad. The keyboard is also small (seven inches wide, six inches high) and requires no complicated installation.

The range of gadgetry available to help the disabled use computers is amazing, and the list grows longer all the time. Brown & Co. of South Hamilton, Massachusetts, for example, has developed a foot-controlled pedal switch that allows the computer to be operated entirely with one hand—the pedal duplicates the appropriate key when two keys (the shift key and a letter key, for instance) need to be activated at once. Another interesting gadget is the Stride NOD, available through Symbiotic Office Systems in Metairie, Louisiana. The NOD translates the movement of a small piece of reflective material into computer-readable information. When it's attached to glasses, for example, a head movement can position the screen cursor.

Among the technological devices for the disabled that have evolved from general-market electronic development is the long-range optical pointer produced by Adaptive Communication Systems in Pittsburgh, Pennsylvania. It's basically a light pen used as a head pointer to operate a standard keyboard. Like a light pen, it can be used as a direct-selection device or as a keyboard emulator.

Another company, American West Engineering, has recently developed a device called MultiMouse. Designed primarily for persons with only one hand (left- and right-handed models are available), its six buttons can emulate all the keys on an IBM keyboard. The MultiMouse sells for less than $300.

Through an arrangement between IBM and Easter Seals initiated in 1988, disabled persons can purchase a range of other helpful devices that work in conjunction with a home computer for a savings of up to 30 to 50 percent off list price. (Call your local IBM or Easter Seals office for up-to-date information about this evolving program.) One of these devices is a monitor that can produce extra-large print on the screen. Another is a "wobble" switch—a long lever that can be toggled to activate keys and move a cursor for people with limited hand use. Still another is a "computer entry terminal" (a special kind of keyboard) designed specifically for use with an optical pointer (or a light pen), or scanned with a wobble switch.

In short, even the severest disability needn't keep you from operating a computer. But don't think that all these gadgets are simply to make programs work. They aren't. Add a few more peripheral devices and your computer can become an invaluable assistant around the house. The Cash III voice-controlled system, for example, lets people with limited or no use of their hands operate the computer and dial the telephone using voice commands. It will also turn pages, turn on lights, or answer the door—all with one voice command to the computer. The complete system in 1986 was expensive ($9,500) but still a small price to pay for such an array of aids in one package, especially considering that the entire computer system (including hard drive and modem) was included in the price.

Enter the robotic age

Robotic devices can be connected to a computer and can perform a variety of tasks. Some can turn pages for you as you read. One, known as the Apprentice II, is a table-top robot that helps you eat, can grab objects within its reach, and inserts disks

Financing

A major concern about computerized or robotic assistive devices for the disabled is their cost. Beneficial as they might be, many disabled people simply can't afford them. The Butler-in-a-Box sells for $1,495. Computer companies themselves recognize that cost can be a prohibitive factor in allowing the disabled access to such gadgets.

But other means of financing computers and related equipment are available. Depending upon the individual situation, a national (or local) organization that deals with your disability may have a grant or low-interest loan program that would help pay for the device or devices you need. The American Foundation for the Blind has begun a low-interest loan fund to help people buy the Personal Reader, for example. Chrysler Corp., too, has established a program to help reduce the cost to the disabled of installing adaptive driving aids in its new cars and trucks. Operated through Chrysler's Physically Challenged Resource Center, the program provides a cash allowance of up to $500 for these devices. Local dealers have full details and program rules available. The National Lekotek Center (headquarters in Evanston, Ill.) offers computer loans to the disabled through its INNOTEK (Innovations in Technology) division.

But the list doesn't stop there. Steven Mendelsohn's 1988 book *Financing Adaptive Technology: A Guide to Sources and Strategies for Blind and Visually Impaired Users* describes several available sources of funding for all disabled people, not just the blind. The book is available in large print, braille, on cassette, and on Apple and IBM floppy disks. It can be ordered directly from Mendelsohn at the address in the appendix.

Direct grants and low-interest loans from federal or state agencies offer another avenue for funding for computer-related purchases. Are you planning to run a business from your bedroom? You might qualify for a Small Business Administration loan to help you get started. Depending on your circumstances, you might be eligible for financing (partial or whole) through the Social Security Administration. See Chapter 4 for more information on this.

The sources are out there. You just need to do the calling and writing to find out what you qualify for.

into a computer drive. It is operated by voice command, keyboard, or any of the other means mentioned above.

Another, the Butler-in-a-Box from Mastervoice in Los Angeles, can do even more. It doesn't just dial the phone and operate lights by voice command; it operates all the electrical appliances and serves as a burglar alarm, too. A small (about twelve inches high, nine inches wide, and three inches deep) computer, it works by recognizing certain voice commands (which you have to teach it, of course) and sending an electrical signal through the house wiring to receivers installed on the appliances.

Meanwhile, although they're still in the experimental stages, some companies are developing personal mobile robots that respond to voice commands. A tremendous amount of development is taking place in this field now, and more will continue throughout the 1990s. Keep a watchful eye out—these devices will help you.

Keeping up with technology

Sometimes the rush of technology is so rapid that it seems impossible to keep up. By the time you buy a tool and learn to use it, a newer and better one has come on the market. Don't let this hold you back from buying what is state-of-the-art now. If you need what's available, get it and use it. Anything that makes life a bit easier for you is worth having, from a simple flexible vinyl straw to drink with to a robot that answers the door.

A number of "miracle" technologies will always be in the experimental stages and, sadly, beyond the financial reach of most of us. But prices come down, and advanced models do eventually become part of our daily lives. Let's face it: from the time a human first picked up a rock to pound against a piece of flint to come up with a sharper knife edge, man has been inventing better, more efficient tools. That development is just happening faster now.

This shouldn't stop you from staying abreast of what's available, especially since it's fairly easy to stay current. A variety of directories is available through various agencies, both private and public. Lifeboat Press, for instance, publishes an *International Directory of Job-Oriented Assistive Device Sources* that is indexed by impaired function, job title, and disability. IBM, too, has published a "Guide to Adaptive Devices, Software, and Services for Special Education, Vocational Education, Vocational Rehabilitation, and Employers" that is free for the asking. Apple Computer Co. in Cupertino, California, has had a special education division since 1985 and it, too, can provide helpful information. And, if you're armed with a computer and modem by this point, check in regularly with the disabilities forum on CompuServe or one of the disabled-oriented bulletin boards for a look at what's new.

Scan catalogs and send away for leaflets, too. It's well worth anyone's while to get a copy of the catalog of Ways & Means, which specializes in helpful devices and gadgets for the disabled, or one of the others like it. It is filled with gadgetry (some of it commonly available anywhere, to be sure) that can be of great help to the disabled. One such device is the Easiwriter, an easily gripped, rounded pyramid-like affair on ball bearings. It holds a ballpoint pen at the correct angle and with the correct amount of pressure to make writing a simpler task for those with hand impairments. A similar but simpler device is the Arthwriter, which is little more than a three-inch plastic ball through which a pen or pencil can be inserted, again making writing a less exacting chore for someone with a hand impairment. It also lists reaching devices, as well as adapters that fit on faucets and door handles to make their operation easier. An "iron guard" designed to guide the free hand and protect it from burns is available for the visually impaired.

Remember, tools like these are devised to assist you in your pursuit of greater activity. Learn what you can about them. You might come across something a friend can use, or you might think of a way to improve on an existing gadget or invent a new one. Few things we come across in life are useless. If we wait long enough, we'll normally find a use for some bit of information which seemed unimportant at the time.

Jon Peterson

Jon Peterson suffers from severe cerebral palsy. C.P. affects people in different ways: speech impediments, lack of motor coordination, or a combination of the two. Some cerebral palsy victims lead fairly normal lives and walk with a slight limp; others are confined to a wheelchair and require a twenty-four-hour-a-day attendant.

Jon was born three months prematurely. Six hours later, he stopped breathing for three to four minutes. "The nurse gave me a shot of adrenalin in my heart to get it going again. My lungs and respiratory system were underdeveloped," he says.

Jon's parents realized by the time he was nine months old that he suffered from some kind of handicap. Doctors told the Petersons that Jon had some brain damage, but they didn't know how much.

"The older I got, the tighter and more spastic my muscles got, so it just got harder for me," he remembers.

Jon, who now works as an instructional aide in special education at San Diego High School, was watching *Omni* on public television one night when the program featured a truck driver with cerebral palsy who had had electrodes implanted near his spine. Electrical stimulation had helped him regain the use of his hand. At the time, St. Barnabas Hospital in New York was the only place in the country doing this experimental surgery. Jon contacted the doctor at St. Barnabas to see what could be done for him.

"The doctor told me that the procedure could help cerebral palsy patients whose limbs were affected, but not their speech," he recalls.

Jon was planning to fly to New York when he heard that Dr. Thomas Waltz, a neurosurgeon at Scripps Clinic in La Jolla, California, was willing to perform the surgery.

The surgery cost $12,500 (80 percent of which was ultimately paid by the Petersons' insurance company) and took two hours. Four electrodes were implanted in Jon's neck and wires were put in his right shoulder. The wires were exposed through the chest so doctors could test which combination worked best.

"The four wires were attached to the four electrodes in my neck. The doctors could have used up to sixteen different combinations to see which electrode stimulated the largest area of the body," Jon says.

A week later, a fifty-minute operation was performed to implant a small receiver in Jon's chest. A "sender" is connected to the electrodes in the back of his neck. This transmitter, powered by a nine-volt battery, has two small dials that regulate the flow of current through the body.

"If I turn the dial up too high, it feels like an electric shock," says Jon. "This is the way it works: the electrical currents are breaking the spasticity. The reason I'm spastic in the first place is that, somehow, the messages between the brain and muscles are out of control. After this procedure, the message from the brain gets to the muscles, which work better. I also have physical therapy to retrain the muscles."

Jon now talks enthusiastically about this new electrical stimulation: "It's helped my circulation. I have more control of my left arm. Now I can grasp things in my left hand and hold onto things. I can stretch my left arm and straighten it out over my head with the hand open. I'm generally much more relaxed. I can also keep my legs apart now; before they would always be tightly together. I don't have as many spasms as I used to."

Jon's story of how electrode implantation helped him is one of a growing number of similar success stories. *Parade* magazine reported in January 1988, for example, that electrical stimulation has enabled five paralyzed husbands to become fathers and that computer-driven electrical stimulation has enabled paraplegics treated at the Veterans Administration Medical Center in Cleveland, Ohio, to walk.

While a discussion of electrode implantation may appear out of place in the gadget chapter of this book, what is implanted in the body is, in the final analysis, actually a "gadget." And, thanks to today's rapid advancements in electronics, semi-conductors, and robotics, medical scientists continue to come up with what can be called orthopedic and muscular miracles.

The best thing to do when you hear or read about something that interests you is track it down to its source. Write or phone the television station, the program, the newspaper, the magazine, or wherever you learned of it. Just remember, if what you're after appeared on radio or TV, write down the specific program and the time and date; if you saw it in a magazine or newspaper, note the date and, if possible, the name of the reporter.

In the case of experimental work like Jon's implant, it is often necessary to track down the hospital and the doctor who does the work. Try the people at your particular disability organization, disease foundation, local hospitals, and the clinics specializing in your problem. All of this may take time, but it's worth it. Jon Peterson started with a story on television and ended up able to use his hands again. Sometimes you'll discover you're chasing a rainbow. Sometimes not. Either way, it's worth the try.

Housing and the disabled

For years, the disabled—especially those in wheelchairs—had to make do with tract homes designed for able-bodied residents. It was frustrating for the disabled to have small bedrooms (which were difficult to turn around in in a wheelchair), narrow doorways, kitchen shelves too high, furniture an obstacle instead of a comfort.

The housing industry has been slow to meet the needs of the disabled, but things are changing, finally. Floor plans are now available for houses with ramps instead of steps, low shelves with Lazy Susans for easy access, special showers and bathtubs for independent bathing.

Many of these unique designs have been created by the disabled themselves. After all, those in wheelchairs are in a prime position to know what's beneficial, what's needed, and what's not. Aulton and Marene Aulger are one such pair. They designed their own 2,500-square-foot home in San Diego.

Built in 1950, theirs was one of the first houses planned to accommodate wheelchairs. The Aulgers, married since 1945, thus truly qualified as pioneers in home design for the disabled. Aulton was paralyzed in a 1940 Navy plane crash; Marene contracted polio when she was twenty-one. Both are paraplegics and both have master's degrees (his in engineering; hers in educational counseling).

Most of the features in their home are their own design. The house has no steps anywhere, only ramps. The rooms are large (the master bedroom sixteen feet square, the family room thirty feet by seventeen feet). The doorways are three feet wide (twenty-eight inches is standard) to accommodate wheelchairs. In the living room, the sofa has built-in end tables so there's no need to worry about bumping into them and knocking them over. In the large family room, two-foot-square tables sit against the wall as decoration, but they fold out on hinges for use as desks, snack tables, or whatever. When not in use, they're out of the way of wheelchairs. Four-foot-wide hallways (instead of the standard three feet) easily accommodate a wheelchair. And, for a flourish, a wine rack is built into a drawer that rolls out on casters—similar to a desk file cabinet. (Outside, sidewalks around the house are extra wide for wheelchairs, and built-in planter boxes are thirty inches high for easy watering and gardening).

In the bathroom, the bathtub side swings open just like a refrigerator door and seals tight when shut. It is one of the few items the Aulgers didn't design. A person in a wheelchair can roll right up to it, slide onto a seat (or use the hydraulic lift), and get into the tub. Safety bars are mounted on one side. Once the "door" is sealed tight, the water is run in. The shower is unique, too. A stainless steel seat swings out and automatically locks in place as a person sits in it. It can then be swiveled or turned to the bather's content while the water sprays merrily away. *Ways & Means* stocks a programmable-memory telephone that can be mounted in the shower as an extra safety precaution.

In the Aulgers' large kitchen all cabinets are thirty-two inches from the floor. The mixer, blender, and ice crusher are mounted in a pull-out drawer for greater stability. Another drawer has a board nailed across the top with large holes in the center. Mixing bowls fit in the holes, again for added stability. The Corningware stove is also thirty-two inches high and easy to clean because of its completely flat cooktop. A large pantry, seven by four by two feet, has a shelved panel that slides out, providing easy access to the rear shelves. The shelves are staggered so that when one shelf is pulled out, items can easily be seen on the others. No can or jar is hidden. Kitchen shelves can be lowered with a motor-driven device for easy reach.

The range of kitchen utensils for the disabled defies description. Mixing bowls with handles are plentiful. Specially designed plates are available in a variety of designs, including one Royal Doulton pattern for formal occasions. *Ways & Means* lists pages of eating utensils, too, in a variety of designs. You can even get an electric corkscrew to open that special bottle of wine you've been saving.

For more information on home design for the disabled, *Housing and Home Services for the Disabled* by Maxine H. Atwater

(Harper & Row, 1977) is recommended. Ms. Atwater can be contacted directly at 500 23rd St., N.W., Suite 308, Washington, D.C. 20037.

Don't forget the simple things

With all the attention being paid to computers, experimental implants, robots, and whatnot, it's easy to forget the simple things—the things we need to get through the days and nights. Because they are considered everyday devices, they usually get ignored. However, because our reliance on them is almost second nature, we can't afford to ignore things like beds, wheelchairs, or lifts.

Beds

The average able-bodied person spends a third of his or her life in bed, and those who are disabled spend even more time than that. It stands to reason we should choose the right one. Some say the only way to find the right bed is to sleep on it, but stores frown on their customers taking a nap in the window display, so here are a few other ways to become knowledgeable enough to pick the right bed for you.

First, consider the firmness of the mattress, the size of the bed, and the ease of maneuverability of the various positions. Sit on the bed, move around on it, and lie down. Bounce up and down on it if you can. Does it hold your weight without sagging? The farther you sink into a mattress, the more difficult it will be for you to move. A too-soft bed may sound luxurious and restful, but it is just the opposite because your muscles have to use more energy to move any part of your body. Can you turn with a minimum of work? Can you sit on the edge without it slanting? Does it hold you steady when you traverse from bed to chair or from lift to bed? Don't hesitate to ask the salesperson for permission to make these experiments.

Consider the size of the room where you'll put the bed, the size of the surface you want, and your own size. Make sure there is adequate room for the wheelchair, lift, or whatever else you need in the bedroom. Next, consider what is going to be on the bed besides you: a telephone, perhaps, or books, magazines, a tea tray, or a teddy bear. Finally, be sure you and the bed are in proportion to one another. A person who stands six feet four and weighs 285 pounds is not going to be happy in a bed suitable for someone five feet two who weighs ninety-five pounds.

Equally important is your ability to electrically control the positions of the bed. Make sure you can easily, with the push of a button or other device, raise the head to a comfortable position. Can you change the knee position? And can you do the same relative to the mattress' distance from the floor? That last question is important, because adjusting the height of the bed from the floor can greatly facilitate your own ability to transfer from bed to gurney, chair, or walker, and it often makes dependence on a lift unnecessary. By simply having the bed at a convenient height, a ninety-year-old paraplegic stroke victim with limited muscular energy can get from bed to chair and back again unaided.

Wheelchairs

Wheelchairs come in as many sizes, designs, and colors as cars these days. With a little hunting, you can find just about anything you could possibly imagine. And if it isn't available "off the rack," you can always have it customized to your personal needs. Special chairs are available for square-dancing, playing basketball, and running the Boston Marathon. Some come fitted with an electric motor, a computerized communication system, and a respiratory device. There's a lightweight, stripped-down version that folds to eleven inches for storage on yachts or airplanes. You can even get one with special wheels for going to the beach.

When shopping for a wheelchair, keep a couple of things in mind: how much actual physical support you need and what you want to do while you are sitting in it besides move.

Your physical condition and life-style should be the two main criteria for choosing a wheelchair. Helynn has always been partial to Everest and Jennings' smallest, lightest-weight, most stripped-down model. It folds compactly and can be tossed easily into a car, boat, plane, or train. Her friends claim she's more interested in a fast getaway than in comfort.

You might think one chair is pretty much like another, but subtle differences from one manufacturer to another can significantly influence your choice. Motions Designs, Inc. (addresses of several wheelchair manufacturers are listed in the appendix), for example, builds an inexpensive, lightweight, small chair with options that include anti-tip tubes, high brake extension handles, grade assistance, leg straps, plastic-coated or projection handrims, tray table, seat belt, seat pouch, backpack, frame-impact guards—and it comes in different colors! It's the wheelchair equivalent of the ten-speed bike.

Kuschall of America builds a side-to-side-folding chair designed so that 70 percent of the chair's weight is positioned over the rear wheels for better balance and handling. Also a portable lightweight, the Champion 2000 has a fold-down back so it can travel in very small spaces—even in the overhead bin on some commercial aircraft. You can add all sorts of things: a seat belt, stroller handle, handrims, crutch holder, amputee axle plate, and so on.

Take your time when choosing a wheelchair. It's as important to you as buying a car is to other people. It is your mode of transportation, and you should have one in which you are comfortable. Investigate thoroughly before buying, and consider a motorized chair. Motorized chairs in particular are becoming more and more popular, especially in cities with curb modifications, ramps, and more accessible buildings. Motorization gives you freedom to go on your own, independent of someone else's schedule.

Lifts

Perhaps the greatest variety of lifts come from Ted Hoyer and Company, Inc., and are distributed by Everest and Jennings. A quick trip through the products in the Hoyer catalog will probably convince you that this company has just about covered the gamut of needed lifting devices: bed to chair, or chair to commode, bathtub, swimming pool, car, and van. But if you need or want to look further, you'll find other manufacturers listed in the appendix.

Different lifts do different jobs, but the accessories are interchangeable. So the same rule applies here as for buying wheelchairs: make sure the lift satisfies your specific needs and wishes before you buy. Start with the basic lift and proceed with whatever expansion program you plan. If you can't get from bed to chair to car on your own, these lifts save your attendant a lot of backache and muscle strain, especially if you are difficult to lift and carry.

The Hoyer Lifter is lightweight and portable. The lift itself weighs only forty-six pounds and fits easily into the back seat or trunk of a standard-size car. A hydraulic jack is standard, but you can have a mechanical jack at an additional cost. This lift can be useful for bed to chair and chair to commode use, as well as wheelchair to car or van. A number of different slings with or without restraint straps are available to go with it.

I-Tec of Huntington Beach, California, builds an overhead track lift called the Independent Transport, which is electrically powered and hand-operated with a switch box. A programmable automatic shut-off and a mechanical stop insure that the unit stops in the proper place. The unit mounts on ceiling tracks or can be free-standing. In some cases it could even eliminate the need for an around-the-clock attendant.

For getting in and out of cars and vans, several types of Kartop Lifts are on the market. These lifts attach securely to the car roof without need for drilling any holes and stack compactly when not in use. Check with Hoyer about the Kartop's requirements to make sure it can be used on your car. Some car and van roofs may not be compatible; it won't work with vinyl tops, for instance. Other companies make van and minibus lifts that consist of platforms onto which you simply wheel yourself. These lifts then rise to the proper height so that you can wheel yourself into the vehicle. This is probably the simplest and most hassle-free type of van lift, especially if you prefer to use a tie-down device to stay in your chair.

Bruno builds the Out-Sider, another design of fully automatic lift: a platform lift attached to the rear of your car that eliminates the need to carry your scooter or chair inside your car. It has an automatic hold-down device for your scooter or wheelchair. Mac's Lift Gate makes a similar lift. You just unlock the control panel with your key, press the button, and it's ready to load. You can enter from either side, so you can't be boxed in.

Still another lift, the Top Cat, puts the wheelchair (folded, of course) on the roof of your vehicle. It's powered by your car's 12-volt battery using a hand control plugged into the cigarette lighter socket. It raises or lowers your chair to the side of the car within easy reach of the driver and without coming into contact with the car.

Several bathtub lifts are available. One (made by Hoyer) uses the standard lifter, but its clamp-on unit cannot be used on roll rim, plastic, or fiberglass tubs. Another, built for those less disabled who want privacy in the bath, offers safe bathing for anyone who can operate the lift without help. The hydraulic lift raises and lowers a person into a standard sixteen- to twenty-inch-high tub. Hoyer also makes the Swimming Pool Lifter for recreational and therapeutic swimming.

One final type of lift cannot be overlooked—the one that carries us upstairs. If you live in a lovely old home in the East or Midwest, or in a second-floor condominium in the Sun Belt, you'll understand the value of a simple platform that ascends a staircase with a seemingly effortless glide. A flight of stairs to the wheelchair-bound can be the perpendicular rock face of Half Dome in Yosemite. Any contraption that can transport you up and down is a thing of joy. Several companies that make stairway lifts are listed in the appendix.

Respiratory aids

Respiratory dysfunction can be caused by birth defects, illnesses, and physical damage from accidents. The need for respiratory aid is vital and cannot prudently be ignored. Nor can it be set aside until later. Thankfully, a few mechanical gadgets now on the market help alleviate the physical and emotional distress caused by insufficient oxygen.

A Warning

Some serious problems can develop gradually if you're not careful.

Helynn's own breathing problem developed so gradually that she was unaware of what was happening—unaware of both the physical and the mental impairment that was occurring. This insidiously slow deterioration is almost impossible for the victim to detect because its development is so gradual. Even the relentless march of the results of blood-gas tests failed to convince Helynn, because the decline of oxygen and the rise of carbon dioxide (CO_2) was spread over a period of four years.

Helynn woke up one morning in an iron lung. Several years later she is still in what she calls her "Yellow Submarine."

For respiratory patients who do not require something as restrictive as an iron lung, the J.H. Emerson Company of Cambridge, Massachusetts, manufactures the "rocking bed." For some, it may seem like riding a Brahma bull or a storm-tossed ocean ferry. Many people, however, swear by it and find its rocking motion both soothing and sleep-inducing.

The continuous motion of the bed keeps circulation active, bowel and bladder functions normal, and diaphragmatic mobility constant. Patient accessibility also means greater independence and simplified nursing procedures. Used mainly at night, these beds operate smoothly, quietly, and reliably. In addition to the standard adult models, junior models are available. Side rails may be added. The adult bed operates on standard house current and comes with a four-inch-thick foam rubber mattress, an adjustable footboard, and a belt guard.

Chest shells are sometimes used in conjunction with iron lungs or rocking beds for daytime assistance and travel, since traveling with either of the bigger items would be nearly impossible. Generally the shell requires a power pack, which is available where you rent or buy the shell. The shells come in a variety of standard, short, half, deep, and long sizes. Designed for comfort, they are lightweight, flexible, and durable. The permanent sponge-rubber seal is covered with soft neoprene for a snug fit. One model, the Huxley Cuirass, will often ventilate patients when others fail because it covers a greater area of the abdomen. A chest shell with straps weighs about ten pounds.

The pulmo-wrap is another type of noninvasive, negative-pressure machine for disabled people to consider. Like other such devices, it has advantages and disadvantages. It consists of an interlocking backplate/grid combination and either a zippered or pullover wrap. The pulmo-wrap offers versatile night, intermittent day, or travel-time ventilation aid. Different styles of pulmo-wraps exist. Two zippered styles offer a full-body enclosure wrap in adult or youth sizes and a short sixty-inch model that is open at the bottom and closes with a belt or loop below the grid. The pullover style may be used as either a half-body or full-body enclosure wrap. In the half-body configuration the pullover wrap allows easy access to personal needs. The fabric of the pulmo-wrap allows X-ray penetration without removal.

The smallest of the ventilation aids is the exsufflation belt, usable for both restrictive and obstructive pulmonary problems. It is lightweight and more comfortable than the other devices described here, but you must be either in a sitting or semi-reclining position for it to work—you can't lie flat to sleep. The belt works by means of intermittent abdominal pressure. Incorporated within a supportive corset, an expandable bladder rhythmically inflates. As this bladder compresses the abdomen, the diaphragm is forced upward. When the bladder deflates, the diaphragm falls to its resting position. The exsufflation belt affords increased freedom and mobility and can be powered by a wheelchair-mounted portable ventilator.

Tying up loose ends

You should, of course, consult the manufacturer of any device you buy to determine what sorts of portable power sources you can use. A variety of charge-retaining, spillproof batteries and accessories are available for portable and emergency ventilators, for example, as well as for other types of medical equipment. One good idea is to keep a sealed, spillproof, deep-cycle marine battery (they have extra-long life and are available at most medical supply stores) for home use in case of power outages or other emergencies. A deep-cycle marine battery can absorb a deep discharge and recharge without damage. A sealed, spillproof battery will prevent acid splashes and boilover and thus prevent damage to you and your ventilator.

Remember, too, that special arrangements are required when traveling by air with ventilators, wheelchairs, and other equipment. Gel cell-type batteries are required on airplanes, for example, according to the "Incapacitated Passengers Air Travel Guide." This publication, available from the International Air Transport Association, Traffic Services Administrator, 200 Pearl St., Montreal, Quebec H3A 2R4, Canada, is a must for disabled travelers and is available at a nominal fee.

Another valuable source of information for respiratory aids, machines, and accessories is Lifecare. The main office is located at 655 Aspen Ridge Dr., Lafayette, Colo. 80026 (303-666-9234). Check to see if an office is near you. Lifecare can supply you extensive helpful information.

As we mentioned earlier, the list of devices available to aid the disabled runs the gamut, from specially designed frisbees and backpacks to sophisticated robotic devices. If you can think of it, chances are someone makes it. If no one does, don't despair. You can probably figure out a way to make it yourself, as David Muir of Irvine, California, did. A quadriplegic because of muscular dystrophy, David was frustrated because he could not find a device to enable him to speak after he had a tracheotomy. He fitted a one-way valve onto his tracheotomy tube and was not only able to speak but also to breathe more naturally. David and Dr. Victor Passy are now distributing the valve.

The trick may be to find it

But you usually don't have to go to such lengths. In this chapter we have just scratched the surface of the kinds of devices technology and human ingenuity have made available. Almost anything you can imagine is out there to help you. The trick, often, is to find it. To do that, start with the appendix at the end of this book. Write postcards to several of the companies and organizations listed there.

Another possibility is to order Dorothy O'Callaghan's catalog of catalogs, a directory of more than 200 mail-order catalogs specializing in the particular needs of the disabled. The chances of finding what you are looking for are pretty high and you might even came across usable items you didn't know were available. The directory costs $2.50 from Dorothy O'Callaghan, P.O. Box 19083, Washington, D.C. 20036.

As you build your network, you'll get more addresses and make more contacts. One other thing's certain, too: you'll have plenty to read.

CHAPTER SIX

Up, Up, and Away

Travel is largely a matter of logistics. You should be pretty expert in logistics by now, so don't let that stop you. Like everything else, planning and preparation well in advance will usually resolve such issues.

Money, however, may be another matter. Nearly everyone who travels faces that issue; it isn't unique to you. A major source of contention among travel companions is often money. Will this trip be first class, tourist, or *wundervogel*? It often becomes a smattering of all three. The disabled person has to decide several things early:

- Where do I want to go?
- How much comfort and physical luxury is necessary or do I want?
- Will it be a package tour or an independent adventure?
- What can I/we afford to spend?

An early decision on anything concerning money is important for your companions' sake, too. They have to budget for the trip, just like you. When you think about travel, remember that a good many of the challenges (they aren't "problems" unless we make them that) of travel are shared by both able-bodied and disabled people. Yet just about everyone can manage, somehow, to go someplace. Put your logistics expertise to work; all you need are your imagination and some planning. And just in case you think none of this is for you, remember that, after you get your degree, you might wind up with a job that will require some business travel. You can prepare for that eventuality now.

Make a list

This chapter is designed to show you how to plan, and enjoy, a major excursion, not to replace any of the dozens of travel guides on the market. First, set up your computer, get out a notepad and pen, or begin musing aloud. You're about to spend a few days of delicious pleasure figuring out how to bring fantasy and reality together. Begin by making a list:

1. Destination
2. Itinerary
3. Money
4. Entourage
5. Medical supplies
6. Legal documents
7. Luggage

You'll identify subheadings under each of these items as you plan. In short order, you'll have a checklist of things you can cross off as you finish them.

Destination

Where in the world do *you* want to go? Let your imagination and your fantasies guide you. Daydream. Quadriplegics with respiratory devices *have* been on the Great Wall of China. Remember the Chinese saying: the journey of a thousand *li* begins with one step. Surely there's a place, a Shangri-la, you've always wanted to see. Write it down. There! You have your destination.

Financial considerations, of course, force us all to think in

Guidebooks

You might not find them in your local bookstore, but several guides designed specifically for disabled travelers are available. For example, Frommer published a *Guide for the Disabled Traveller* in 1984; the book covers travel in the United States, Canada, and Europe and includes lists of accessible hotels and restaurants. The U.S. Government Printing Office has publications ranging from air travel to camping (*Travel Tips for the Handicapped and Access Travel: Airports* and *Camping in the National Park System*), with several others in between. Contact your nearest Government Printing Office branch or write to the Consumer Information Center, Pueblo, Colo. 81009. *Consumer Information About Air Travel for the Handicapped* is available from Trans World Airlines (605 Third Ave., New York, N.Y. 10016). Other airlines also publish information concerning disabled travel. Call the local airline office or your travel agent to request information.

The National Center for a Barrier-Free Environment (8401 Connecticut Ave., N.W., Washington, D.C. 20015) prints *A List of Guidebooks for Handicapped Travellers*, and the May 1984 issue of *Paraplegia News* describes nine publications that deal with travel for the disabled, including guides to Amtrak and bus travel in the U.S. In addition, a number of resource guides for disabled travelers are available. "LTD Travel" (116 Harbor Seal Court, San Mateo, Calif. 94404) is a newsletter for disabled travelers that includes regularly updated information about travel agents for the disabled. *Handi-Travel: A Resource Book for Disabled and Elderly Travellers* is a comprehensive guide for people whose disabilities include mobility, hearing, and sight impairments. It is available from the Canadian Rehabilitation Council for the Disabled, Suite 2110, One Yonge St., Toronto, Ontario, Canada M5E 1E5.

practical terms. Perhaps Vienna is your Shangri-la, but your bankroll is only a thousand dollars. Can you do it? Yes, but it will take you a little longer. Give yourself enough advance time to save the money, or come up with a way to earn some extra. The point is, as with anything else, to identify the goal, then determine what you have to do to achieve it.

Once you've chosen a destination, set about assembling all the

Two Travel Agents

Betty Hoffman, a feisty travel agent in her eighties, has paved the way for many disabled travelers. In 1959 she helped three disabled people make a trip to Hawaii, and she's been in business ever since.

Betty, disabled herself from "a couple of strokes" and "in a wheelchair for some time," has taken disabled tour groups to nearly every country in the world. Her groups have toured Afghanistan, Nepal, Iraq, Israel, Turkey, Poland, Europe, Asia— even Iran three times. Betty now runs Evergreen Travel (4114 198th St. SW, Lynnwood, Wash. 98036; phone 1-800-435-2288 or [206] 776-1184) and has taken "all types" of disabled on tours.

"We visit areas not considered wheelchair-accessible. We take railroad trips, climb flights of stairs in European castles and museums, and go jet-boating up white-water rivers," she says. "Over the years, our disabled have gone sightseeing on elephantback, have toured the ruins of Machu Picchu, have traveled by gondola in Venice, and ascended the Great Wall of China. We make the impossible possible."

She sends each tour member a questionnaire first to find out

ingredients that go into savoring that destination. It's not complicated. Contact the tourist information office for the destination you've chosen. Most foreign countries maintain such offices in the United States; several have more than one. Addresses can be found at the conclusion of this book; you'll also find them in travel guides.

On the subject of travel guides, now is a good time to look at one or more of the many travel guides available for virtually every destination in the world. Get them from your local library. You'll want to buy one or more later, but for now, just scan a few to get an idea of your destination. Look at both the travel guides and photo books. They'll provide helpful tips as well as whet your appetite.

If you're traveling in the United States, contact chambers of

what limitations exist. Depending on the limitations of the partici-
pants, the group may be as small as fifteen or as large as thirty. Her
agency conducts eight to ten tours a year for people in wheelchairs.

Wes Johnson is also a wheelchair-bound travel agent. A truck
accident in 1980 paralyzed him from the waist down. Before the
accident, the thirty-one-year-old graduate of San Diego State University had been a member of a Navy helicopter rescue team. His
career today grew out of his frustration at trying to travel on his
own in his wheelchair. Now he helps other disabled people travel
and works to make the travel industry more sensitive to the needs
of the disabled. His agency is Uni-Globe Wide World Travel, 3683
Midway Dr., Suite G, San Diego, Calif. 92110; phone (619)
225-9744.

Wes advises several companies that work with wheelchair travelers. He also arranges individual packages for wheelchair travelers
who prefer to travel independently. He cautions that getting from
airport to hotel (or elsewhere) can be a problem. "Very few taxis or
buses have lifts for electric wheelchairs," he says. "There are
beautiful hotels all over the world, completely set up to accommodate wheelchairs, but the biggest problem for the disabled traveler,
often, is getting to them." Checking with the hotel ahead of time
about transportation can solve this problem.

commerce for cities on your itinerary and the department of
tourism for states you plan to visit. Explain when you plan to be
there and ask for information about anything that's on your mind:
accommodations, car rental, rail travel. Be sure to request information about special access for the disabled. You'll get back a
large package of brochures and maps that will keep you busy for
days.

Itinerary

Now it's time to figure out how to get where you want to go.
You can do it one of two ways: call a travel agent or do it yourself.
The first is easier, certainly, although it robs you of the chance to
savor the anticipation. Besides, even if you do make some or all of

your arrangements through a travel agent, you'll still need to do some planning: dates of departure, destination, special requirements, accommodation, car rental, and so forth.

Travel Agents. A number of travel agencies specialize in arrangements for disabled travelers. Most major cities have at least one. Check your local Yellow Pages; some agencies advertise the fact that they arrange trips for the disabled. If you don't find anything there, however, call a few travel agencies; that could yield someone in your area. For a more structured approach, contact the Travel Information Center at Moss Rehabilitation Hospital, 12th Street and Tabor Road, Philadelphia, Pa. 19141, (215) 329-5715. This agency doesn't plan trips or make reservations, but it will share what information it has about an area along with sources of other general information helpful to disabled travelers. Some of the information comes from previous users of the service. Another possible source of travel agents and information is the Society for the Advancement of Travel for the Handicapped, 26 Court St., Suite 1110, Brooklyn, N.Y. 11242, (718) 858-5483. Mobility International (P.O. Box 3551, Eugene, Ore. 97403, [503] 343-1284) deals with international educational exchange and recreational travel. *Itinerary* (P.O. Box 1084, Bayonne, N.J. 07002, [201] 858-3400) is a bimonthly magazine specializing in accessible travel.

In 1984, Murray Vidockler from the Society for the Advancement of Travel for the Handicapped predicted that within a few years disabled travelers would represent a $30-billion market. While that tremendous amount of money may seem improbable, it has undoubtedly contributed to the increased number of travel agencies specifically designed to help disabled travelers see the world. Many have begun to specialize according to disability or destination—like Palex Tours (P.O. Box 33015, Haifa 31033, Israel), which deals exclusively with tours of Israel for the disabled.

Do It Yourself. Making your own travel arrangements isn't as hard as you might think. Start with a map. Locate your Shangri-la. Figure out how you're going to reach it: land, sea, air, or perhaps all three. Determine how long you'll stay and select your departure and return dates. Allow yourself as much advance planning time as possible—two or three months if you can, more if you need additional time to accumulate money. You'll be writing various places for rates and information about accessibility. Finally you'll pick a hotel and send a deposit. Then you'll wait for confirmation. All that correspondence will probably take four to six weeks, at least. Helynn and her attendant, Wilma, spent nearly a year in preparation for a trip to England. They reserved hotels, rented a camper, and arranged to spend a week on a canal boat. Once they arrived, the rest was comparatively easy.

Next, spend some time on the telephone. Call the airlines' toll-free numbers (they're listed in the back of this book, and many are in the Yellow Pages). Tell the reservation agent where you want to go and when. Identify precisely your special needs— oxygen, wheelchair, special accessibility, or whatever—and specifically request the *lowest available fare*. Airlines maintain a confusing array of fares, so you must ask for the "lowest available fare" to get the best deal. Next, ask about lower fares if you travel on dates other than the ones you've chosen. Most airlines, for example, have Monday-through-Thursday excursion fares; the price goes up on Friday. Most of us would gladly leave on vacation a day early to save fifty to a hundred dollars or more. Finally, ask about any extra charges for special services, departure taxes, and other hidden costs. Write this information down.

"Airlines have come a long way toward accommodating the wheelchair traveler," Wes Johnson, himself a wheelchair-bound travel agent, says. One organization that has helped this progress is Access to the Skies, a group of paralyzed veterans who work to eliminate obstacles and standardize air travel for the disabled. A government regulation now requires that airlines allow dogs with blind travelers, for example.

Oxygen is now available on many flights, too, as long as the airline has advance notice. When you make your reservations, ask about the company's policy on oxygen. Use the answer as one of the criteria for selecting an airline. Airline policies toward this vital commodity are in a state of flux, and so is the charge for the service. It's a step in the right direction and, for those with respiratory problems, a most welcome one. Since oxygen helps overcome fatigue, it could be especially helpful for those who tire easily on, say, a long overseas flight. If a few dollars can offset exhaustion and alleviate some of the effects of jet lag, the money is well spent.

Johnson ranks American Airlines as the best for wheelchair travelers. "It's the most consistent," he says. "United Airlines is also good." But he sees some glaring omissions by the airlines: "The blind are not told where the emergency exits are; the directions should be printed in braille. Flight attendants should give their instructions in sign language, too. And the instructions should also be written for the hearing-impaired."

Don't make a reservation yet. Prices vary widely, so keep calling. Keep a list, and compare. Weigh the lowest fare with the convenience and the availability of the assistance you need. *Then* decide. You'll have done essentially what travel agents do, but you'll have the satisfaction of doing it yourself—and you'll probably learn some things in the bargain.

Now go back to the map on which you originally marked your Shangri-la. Make a short list of the things you need to do to get where you want to go—air travel, car rental, rail passes, advance hotel reservations, and so forth.

Say you live in St. Louis, Missouri, and you want to go to Quebec, Canada. All you need to arrange is for a friend to drive you to the airport, catch a plane, and pick up a car in Quebec. But if you live in Salt Lake City and want to view the ruins of Machu Picchu in Peru, you have to get to the airport, change planes in Los Angeles, fly Peru Air, hire a cab in Lima, take a train, and—if all goes well—arrive at that very mysterious spot.

When you select your modes of transportation (not just for the main journey, but once you've arrived) note the special help you'll need boarding and disembarking and estimate the time this is likely to take. Figure out how you're going to get on and off these assorted vehicles. You may long to ride through London on the upper deck of one of those gorgeous red double-deck buses, but climbing a narrow, winding staircase while it's moving may pose a problem. Still, with a little advance planning, certain obstacles can be surmounted.

Transportation over water is another ballgame. If you don't

suffer from a fear of drowning just because you can't swim and are weighted down with braces and harnesses, a boat is a delightful way to travel. Nothing equals it for sheer luxury. Everything is on board and right at hand. All you need to do is eat, lean back, and watch the clouds overhead.

Obviously, white-water rafting on the Snake River is different from a Caribbean cruise. But you actually can do both. The contrast would give you something to talk about for years. Some ships cruise the inland waterway to Alaska, where the scenery is spectacular. Some ships go through the Panama Canal. (Richard Halliburton swam it accompanied by a rowboat, but we don't recommend that even though it's unbelievably cheap—use of the canal is charged by the ton!) Some ships tour the fjords of Norway; others traverse the Mediterranean. Cruise ships go everywhere. One other beauty of cruises is that the price includes cruise, meals (normally about six a day), and stateroom.

More and more cruise lines are offering trips for the disabled, and you can also travel on "regular" cruises. Holland America Line, for instance, has added wheelchair accessible cabins to three of its ships; another of its large ships, the *Rotterdam*, is popular among disabled travelers because of its large staterooms and its wheelchair-accessibility. Cunard Lines has three wheelchair-accessible ships and Princess Cruises has two, as do Admiral Cruises and Kloster Cruise, Ltd. Royal Cruise Line has one accessible ship.

Money

You might wonder why this category isn't at the top of the list—or at the bottom. After all, travel costs money; the farther you go, the more it costs. But if you put money at the top of your list, you might spend so much time worrying about where to get it that you'll never leave the house. On the other hand, if you put it at the bottom, you might ignore the reality of finances and plan an extravagant itinerary that is impossibly expensive.

Neither of these approaches is particularly unique—to the disabled or the able-bodied. Many people we all know have never traveled because they thought they couldn't afford it. They've spent their vacations dispiritedly, hanging around the house, watching

TV, brooding, and barbecuing in the backyard—all things they've ordinarily done. We've put money in the middle of this list to help you keep it in its proper perspective.

How much money you'll need, of course, depends on where you're going, for how long, how limiting your disability is, and what you plan to do. Only you can identify those things. The planning is the key. If you've decided on a package tour, certain necessary expenses (airfare, lodging, perhaps some meals, airport transfers) are taken care of in advance. The advantage, clearly, is the simplicity. Write one check, and all you have to worry about are incidentals: rental-car cost, other transportation, a few meals, spending money, and souvenirs. Since most of these preset jaunts are double-occupancy, you and your attendant get a good deal. In the end, you'll find that a Caribbean holiday or a week in Hawaii isn't as prohibitive as you'd thought. After the initial cost, additional expenses depend only on your fancy and your cash flow.

Even if you decide to "play it by ear" (take your chances on finding hotels and such once you arrive), there's still good reason to start your planning early. Veteran travelers know that the earlier they buy (and pay for) their plane tickets, the cheaper they usually are. Airfares fluctuate wildly during the year. Cool-weather destinations command higher fares in the summer; warm-weather spots are more expensive in the winter. Therefore, if you're planning a trip to Europe in June, you'll be traveling in what is called peak season. But if you buy, *and pay for*, your tickets the preceding December, you can save as much as $400.

A bit of judicious thought should reveal how much you can comfortably afford. Make sure you're realistic in your calculations. Check one of the guidebooks and determine the approximate per-person cost of accommodations. Write that figure down. Next, check for sample meal prices. Come up with an average cost for breakfast, lunch, and dinner, and write that down. Now list daily transportation costs (taxis, buses, subways, rental cars). Figure in admissions to museums, galleries, and the like. Add those numbers together, then add 15 percent to allow for price increases or other contingencies. Multiply that times the days you'll be gone, and you'll have an approximation of what you need.

If your resources don't add up to what you need, you have some choices. Ask yourself some realistic questions:

- Can you save some money by adjusting your choice of hotel? One great option has been popular for decades in other parts of the world and has enjoyed a recent surge in popularity in the United States: the bed-and-breakfast guest house. You stay in (usually) a refurbished older home, and breakfast is included in the price of your room. Thousands of visitors to Europe—the authors included—can attest to the wonderfully comfortable, pleasant atmosphere in these places (they are everywhere in Europe). Their rates can be as little as one-third the price of a first-class hotel, too. Remember, B & B means *bed and breakfast*. If you've planned on even a moderately priced hotel, you might save money in the long run by staying at B & Bs to eliminate the breakfast expense.

- Do you really need to rent a car? In some places the answer is yes; in others you can get along quite nicely (perhaps better) with public transportation. If you do want to rent, however, you'll have a hard time finding cars with hand controls. Inquire about this and any other special considerations ahead of time. If you're going to Oahu, Hawaii, you might want to rent a car for a day or two to see the island (once you arrive, shop the Yellow Pages for "rent-a-wreck" establishments; despite the names, the cars are well cared for and half the price). In Paris or Amsterdam, you're probably better off with public transportation or taxis. Study your map and check your guidebooks for help.

- Have you read or heard of any travel passes that could save on transportation? Many metropolitan areas offer long-term bus, train, and subway passes that save substantial amounts of money. London Transport, for example, sells a seven-day travel pass for underground and bus travel anywhere in central London for about nine U.S. dollars. (Buy it there; travel agents here will try to sell you the more expensive Explorer pass.) It pays for itself in two or three days. Most nations sell seven- and fourteen-day rail passes that must be purchased before you leave the United States. The best-known is the

Eurail Pass, but individual countries have their own, too. They can cut the cost of train travel by more than half.

♦ Finally, do you need to scale down the trip? Most of us, disabled and nondisabled alike, plan to do too much, anyway, when we visit a new place. Consider your health realistically and be certain that you will be well rested when you embark on your sightseeing adventures. You don't want to spend day after day rushing to stay on a schedule you can't possibly meet. So if you can't make the money balance, consider eliminating a side trip or two.

Still short of cash? Don't despair. There's another approach that is economical and rewarding at the same time. Consider attending the summer session of a college or university in the area you want to visit. In most of the world you can enroll in anything from week-long seminars to eight-week courses and, for one price, live in a dormitory and get three meals a day. If you're working toward a degree, you can probably arrange for at least some transfer credit, and that would mean at least a portion of your travel expenses might be tax-deductible. Even more appealing, many institutions have scholarship or grant money available to help defray your expenses. Summer study is particularly attractive outside the U.S., and the concept sends thousands of students and teachers heading for airports every June. Foreign institutions like the University of London offer an incredible smorgasbord of seminars for visiting students. Besides an exciting learning environment, you'll spend your spare time with people from all over the world. For information on overseas study, contact the Institute of International Education (890 United Nations Plaza, New York, N.Y. 10017). Within the United States, contact directly the colleges and universities in the cities you plan to visit.

Whether you prepay for your trip, pay as you go, or—as the saying goes—"fly now, pay later," no matter how thoroughly you may have checked and rechecked your expense list, it won't be 100 percent accurate; that alone is reason enough to always travel with a credit card or two. Another reason is that, especially in the United States, you'll have difficulty renting a car without a credit card. Two different cards are better than one because not all are accepted everywhere. Look carefully into the types of credit cards available to you. Be sure to check and compare the amounts of the annual fee, the cost just to have the card. Shop for the lowest interest rate, too. Like airfares, interest rates vary drastically.

If you are traveling overseas, American Express is an especially valuable card to carry. American Express offers its members a number of important services worldwide: you can receive mail and emergency messages, change currency, buy traveler's checks, cash a personal check drawn on your home bank, even pay your bill. Note one thing about the American Express card, however: the total balance is due each month.

Along with credit cards, you should look into traveler's checks. They are safer than cash and almost as acceptable. Some small stores and restaurants don't like to accept them because of the paperwork involved (on their part, not yours; all you do is sign them). But hotels and banks will readily exchange them for currency. In a foreign country, you'll often receive a slightly better exchange rate with traveler's checks than with hard cash. Some advocate buying traveler's checks in the currency of the country you're visiting before you leave. While that's more convenient than changing money immediately after a ten-hour plane ride, you'll pay 5 to 10 percent above the exchange rate to get them before you leave. That, compared to the improved rate you can get changing traveler's checks over to currency, makes carrying U.S.-dollar traveler's checks abroad a slightly better, though slightly less convenient, bargain. Whichever approach you take, and wherever you're going, buy some traveler's checks whenever you manage to save a bit of cash. By the time Helynn and her attendant got to England, they had enough British pounds to cover their expenses for five weeks—all accumulated over the course of a year. By saving the money slowly they scarcely felt the drain on their daily resources. It was an almost painless way of putting together the money for the trip.

Be sure you have enough money to guarantee you a safe and comfortable trip, but don't worry yourself needlessly about money. There's no reason to be foolhardy, but don't become preoccupied. Remember, you are going on a trip to experience new adventures. Keep that foremost in your planning.

Entourage

If you aren't compatible with those around you, it doesn't matter where you go or how much money you spend; your trip will not be a success. The wrong companions can ruin the best-planned vacation, and the right companions can turn even a disaster into an exciting adventure.

Compatibility is crucial on a trip. You're all together twenty-four hours a day in unfamiliar circumstances, encountering unexpected setbacks, unfamiliar food, pubs that close at odd hours, buses you can't board, and absurd language misunderstandings, among other things. In the final analysis, patience, compatibility, and a sense of humor are imperative. A strong back really counts, too, when you are choosing your companions.

The number of people you need depends primarily on how much actual physical help you're going to need. First, consider the nursing care you need or are accustomed to. If you have or require an around-the-clock attendant, that person becomes a logical companion. If you don't require a twenty-four-hour attendant, perhaps you can locate attendants through referral agencies in the area you're visiting. Even if your regular full-time attendant is unable to go with you for some reason, you shouldn't despair. Your local referral service may be able to help you find an attendant who will assist you in exchange for travel costs. Various travel agents who arrange trips for the disabled will also have contacts; don't be afraid to ask. Also, contact the Information Center for Individuals with Disabilities (Fort Point Place, First Floor, 27-43 Wormwood St., Boston, Mass. 02110; [617] 727-5540). This organization maintains information on organizations that specialize in travel for disabled tourists. The point is that many possibilities exist. A little perseverance and you can find what you need or want.

The next consideration is the help you need getting on and off vehicles and transporting a wheelchair or orthopedic equipment as well as your luggage. If you plan your own trip and your transportation scheme is varied, two attendants are a good idea. If it is a package tour, find out from the tour director what is recommended for travelers with your specific disability. On a cruise, for example, you may only need one attendant.

Whatever the number you require and however long the trip, draw your companions into the planning and decision-making process. They're going to be part of this adventure, too. A companion for a trip to England will appreciate a role in the planning if, say, he or she wants to trace family history. And if someone on the safari is even partially bilingual, that's an obvious plus in a foreign country. Although most educated people the world over speak some English, many others do not.

Don't ask anyone if they would like to go with you until you decide on where you are going and what you want to do and see when you get there. Be judicious in your choice of fellow adventurers. A particular friend who loves white-water rafting may not be excited about tramping around the art galleries and churches of Florence. Ask among your friends about their experiences on previous vacations. It's the best way to learn their likes and dislikes.

Medical supplies

If you are taking any prescription drugs, be sure to carry with you the amount you will need for the duration of the trip. Tell your doctor your plans and ask for enough medication to carry you through. It wouldn't hurt to have a bit extra in case of delays en route, either.

If you're going to one or more foreign countries, be sure of two things: that the name of the drug is clearly indicated on each bottle and that the countries you enter allow the importation of that particular drug. On rare occasions, you may run into a difficult border crossing. Phone a country's local consul general before you go and ask if your drugs are passable. It can save a lot of grief later on.

It's also a good idea to wear a Medic Alert bracelet or necklace. The Medic Alert Foundation is a highly regarded nonprofit foundation begun by Dr. Marion C. Collins to provide fast, accurate, vital medical information to doctors, paramedics, and others first on the scene of an accident. The Medic Alert caduceus symbol on the face of the tag is recognized worldwide. The other side lists your medical problems and any allergies or reactions to various medicines as well as a toll-free number (in the U.S.) that can be called for a detailed account of your specific needs. This medical information is as important to you in the U.S. as it is in foreign countries—especially for emergency center and trauma ward teams in case of accident or loss of consciousness. An initial fee covers the wearer for life.

For more information concerning this valuable item, phone or write the Medic Alert Foundation International, Turlock, Calif. 95381-1009 (1-800-432-5378 [1-800-ID ALERT]). Information can be updated any time. When you're traveling, it can be the most valuable piece of medical information you carry.

Bear in mind that any gadget that screws into or onto another gadget can also present a problem, particularly in a foreign country. Helynn learned this firsthand with a portable oxygen tank. Boots Chemists is a chain of well-equipped pharmacies in England, but neither Boots nor anyone else in the United Kingdom could refill her tank. The threads on the screws did not match (remember, most of the world uses the metric system). Nowhere was there an adaptor that would bridge the difference. She ended up buying a British-made tank, an extra expense she hadn't counted on.

Be sure to list all the medical and personal care items you might need, such as elimination bags and so forth. If you can't do without it or "jerry-rig" it from something else, take it along. If you need it for medical or personal care, be sure you have it with you. You want to be comfortable physically. If you are not comfortable, how can you enjoy Mona Lisa's smile in the Louvre or the magnitude of the Lincoln Memorial in Washington, D.C.? Above all, though, don't get caught short of medical supplies.

Legal documents

You need to carry a number of papers with you when traveling, especially outside the United States. Among them are medical instructions, credit cards, and a passport with any visas you need.

GPO Catalogs

Two Government Printing Office catalogs list all publications related to travel that can be purchased from the GPO. The catalogs, *Customs, Immunization, and Passport Publications* and *Travel and Tourism,* are available through branch GPO bookstores or can be ordered from the Superintendent of Documents, U.S. Government Printing Office, Washington, D.C. 20402; (202) 783-3238.

As soon as you decide on your destination and the route you will be taking, begin gathering the necessary documents.

The first thing you'll need is your birth certificate. If you don't already have one, write to the Bureau of Vital Statistics in your home state. This can be in one of two places, depending on the state in which you were born. Your birth will have been recorded at the courthouse in your native county; it will also have been recorded at the state capital. If you can't find it in one, try the other. There is a slight charge for the service; it takes time as well.

Even if you're only traveling in the United States, having a passport is a good idea. For one thing, it's the ultimate form of identification. For another, it's good for ten years. Once the travel bug has bitten you, you can cross one item off your next itinerary. After your birth certificate arrives, call your nearest post office and find out what hours they are open for passport applications. You'll need your birth certificate, two two-inch-square photographs, a current photo-identification card, a completed application, and forty-two dollars. Processing usually takes six to eight weeks, but in May the wait is longer because so many students and teachers travel overseas during the summer. If you're traveling abroad, check a travel guide to see if a visa is required for the countries you plan to visit. Then you're almost ready.

Ask your doctor to write a letter describing your physical and medical problems. Ask him to include an account of what medicines he has used to treat you and the schedule he has recommended for you. If you have to visit a doctor on your trip, he or she will appreciate the information. Knowing what medicines you are accustomed to can be vital, especially if substitutions are neces-

---

Help While Abroad

If you're worried about maintaining a link with the United States while you're traveling abroad, remember that there's a U.S. embassy or consulate in most major cities (except for the few countries with which the U.S. does not have diplomatic relations, of course). You can get its address from the State Department (or even some travel guides) before you go, or you can look it up in the phone book once you arrive.

The Overseas Citizen Services branch of the State Department is responsible for activities relating to the protection and assistance of U.S. citizens abroad. It provides help in the event of an arrest, the death of a U.S. citizen, conservation of his/her personal estate abroad, and the repatriation to the U.S. of destitute or ill citizens. This agency also provides a number of other specific services related to U.S. citizens abroad. For further information, contact Overseas Citizen Services, Bureau of Consular Affairs, Department of State, 2201 C St., N.W., Room 4800, Washington, D.C. 20520; (202) 632-3816.

---

sary. Your companions are relieved from the fear of giving any wrong information, too. Most important, your doctor's written instructions and your Medic Alert bracelet are important if you are rendered unable to communicate for any reason. Just remember, an emergency can't be predicted, but its impact can be lessened by a bit of cautious preparation.

Finally, once you have your credit cards and your itinerary is set, ask American Express to send you the addresses of their offices in cities you'll be passing through. Photocopy the list and give it to your friends and family along with an approximate schedule—they can then write to you.

It is important to keep these documents well protected and with you at all times. If any of them are lost, notify the appropriate authorities immediately. Prompt action can save a lot of grief and hassle.

Luggage

Luggage is the bane of every traveler's life. The pitfalls we encounter dealing with it are numerous.

The first trap to avoid is taking too much. Most travel guides will give you packing tips; take their advice. Packing with economy is doubly important for the disabled. Because of the need for medical supplies and mechanical equipment, the disabled generally require more things. Take comfort from the fact that the chances of running into a life-threatening problem are practically nil, especially in Europe, in English-speaking countries, or within the United States. But the probability of minor irritations is fairly high. So if you're addicted to some particular little creature comfort—if it's important to you—take it along. It may be something as minor as your favorite instant coffee. Just remember that you're taking a trip, not moving.

Luggage, by its mere existence, is a nuisance. For one thing, it has to be transported. Which means someone has to transport it. Luggage also has a tendency to get lost or stolen. Then it has to be found. Although airlines get the brunt of lost-luggage jokes, they are not the only culprits. There are also trains, buses, boats, safari porters, and travelers. Travelers themselves misplace or forget as much luggage as anyone else does.

The fewer the boxes, bags, cases, and shoulder bags you have, the less you'll have to absent-mindedly abandon. And the less money you'll have to shell out in tips to various porters. Also, if you are in a wheelchair, you don't want so many bags piled on your lap that you can't see where you are going.

As you prepare, consider what supplies you need to last you safely for the duration of the trip—especially medical supplies, as already discussed. The answer to this varies significantly from individual to individual. Only you and your medical team can make an intelligent decision.

Here are a couple of tips that might get you out of the baggage claim area quicker:

First, if a medicine must be taken at regular intervals, never assume you can buy it in another city. When it is vital to your well-being, carry it with you. That's what hand luggage is for. Don't trust it to checked luggage, especially if you are going to a foreign country. Eliminate glass bottles; they break easily and weigh far more than plastic. Whenever possible, get your medicine in powder or tablet form to avoid spilled liquids. Keep necessary liquids in sealable plastic bags. A leaking bottle of anything can be a real disaster. Don't ruin your vacation by being paranoid about your medicine; just be sensible.

Second, consider using the simple attaché case for your suitcase, especially for trips of two weeks or less. Yes, it's small. Yes, that means you won't carry as much clothing with you (although some inexpensive models seem like small suitcases). And, yes, it fits under an airline seat, so you can have all your belongings with you all the time. It's easy to carry and, if you follow the tips of seasoned travel writers (such as carrying lightweight clothing), it won't be too heavy. The chances of losing it are practically nil.

Helynn went to England for five weeks with only a wheelchair, a portable oxygen tank, and an attaché case. In the case were wash-and-wear dresses, cotton undershirts (for wearing under her back brace), underwear, nylon stockings, an extra pair of ballet slippers, a dark blue twin-sized bedsheet, two ballpoint pens, notepaper, two paperback books, and medicines. Every country has laundromats, and many hotels will do your laundry overnight.

After you've taken care of the medical and the hand-carried attaché case, go over your entire itinerary again and think about what else you might possibly need. If you're going overseas, for example, be sure you've checked out the electric current. Not all countries operate on the same electrical voltage, but you can get adapters at travel or electrical shops at home that will transform the current flow to match your appliance without burning it out. You'll need these adapters for everything from respirator to electric razor and hair dryer.

Above all, don't short-change yourself with things important to your health and comfort. But leave the extras at home. And if you arrive and find you need something you've left at home, consider it an excuse to buy something new.

Wherever you go, adventure awaits you

Thus far, much of what we've discussed has at least implied foreign travel. But traveling within the United States can be just as adventurous, stimulating, and challenging. You can roam the streets of Constitution-era Philadelphia, savor the delights of San Francisco, or stroll through the French Quarter in New Orleans. If the outdoors entices you, you can go hiking in Yosemite National Park, ride the rapids of the Colorado River, or go beachcombing in Hawaii. Several groups arrange regular "adventure vacations" for the disabled; the addresses of some are listed in the appendix.

Besides the obvious advantages of language and general familiarity, traveling in the United States offers additional transportation options. Trains cross the nation daily. Amtrak service has been upgraded steadily in recent years; trains now are more comfortable and frequent than in the recent past. Amtrak coaches are generally accessible for the disabled, and a cross-country train ride is a leisurely reminder of a once-luxurious means of transportation. Taking the train means avoiding the hassle of crowded airports and, once aboard, you can sit back with a good book or relax and watch the countryside glide by. If your destination is within the United States—or even if you find yourself traveling on business from time to time—compare Amtrak prices (the toll-free number is listed in your phone book's white pages) with the airlines. You might be pleasantly surprised.

If you decide to tour the U.S. or Canada by car, some additional considerations are in order. All are small points, certainly, but as veteran traveler Marene Aulger notes, each can save you time and trouble. First of all, have your car thoroughly checked before you leave. Make sure it is in good running condition. Next, if you don't already have one, get one of those windshield shades with the words PLEASE CALL POLICE on one side, just in case your car breaks down in a remote area.

Try to select a motel or hotel with a dining room or adjacent café. Then it won't be necessary to get back in your car to get something to eat. If you are staying in a hotel where an attendant parks your car, be sure to caution him not to touch your hand controls. Finally, always carry a jug of water.

Tip: Get a street map of the city you want to visit. If it's a major foreign center, a map probably came with the information from the country's tourist bureau. If not, try your local bookstore or the American Automobile Association, if you're a member. Study it carefully before you go and, when you get there, you'll be at least roughly familiar with the lay of the land.

Mark three or four likely hotels or B&Bs with pins so you can see their locations at a glance. Write to them, explain your situation, and give travel dates. Ask about rates, wheelchair accessibility, availability of ground-floor rooms (don't say "first floor"; in some countries, that's one floor up from ground level), private baths or proximity of bathrooms, number of steps up from the sidewalk to the entrance, and anything else you think you might need to know.

Another alternative, depending upon the size of your entourage and your spirit of adventure, is to rent a camper or motor home. At home or abroad, these vehicles have the advantage of minimizing the amount of actual moving in and out you have to do to get to bed while being generally reasonable in cost. You don't have to worry about check-out times or going to a breakfast room in the morning. You can move on as the mood strikes you, and campground fees are inexpensive.

Where have you been, and how did you like it?

After you've decided where you want to go, list the places you've already been. Start with the time before you were disabled (if there was a time when you weren't), but be sure to include travel after you became disabled. Don't omit local outings; they are as important to your mobility factor as the longer jaunts.

Add two subheadings (call them "virtues" and "problems," if you like) for each place you listed. First, identify the things that appealed to you most about the place: activities you enjoyed, food you liked, scenery you remember. Then list problems you remember or that you associate with that destination, disability-related or not. They could range from consistently late trains and buses to lack of wheelchair access for tourist attractions. When you're done you'll have a better perspective on your proposed destination as well as a list of factors to consider in making final plans.

Traveling with a Disabled Child

Traveling with a disabled child does not present any problems that differ significantly from any other travel with children. First, the daily medical routine should be adhered to as closely as possible, of course. Extra time should be set aside for rest periods to minimize the depletion of energy; when youngsters are excited about a venture, they are often reluctant to slow down, so it falls to the parents to call a halt from time to time.

Children, like adults, can become a bit disoriented or confused when everything is strange and new. To alleviate some of this feeling, take along a few favorite items. A stuffed animal, a game, a favorite storybook all carry a sense of home and the familiar. Also, all children (like most adults) like to know in advance what is going to happen next and where they are going. Thus it's important to let them in on the plans and listen to their desires and suggestions.

Parents shouldn't hesitate to venture out with a disabled child. Chances are they'll see the world in colors brighter than ever. All the adventure takes is careful preparation and common sense.

Look again at that list of places you've been. Calculate your longest trip in both distance and time. Answer some important questions:

- Did you have enough people along to help you, or too few?
- How did your assorted equipment and gadgetry perform while you were away from home?
- Are more up-to-date, lighter-weight versions available that you can afford?
- Did you need everything?

Sometimes your destination and what you want to do there have to be figured into these calculations. Keep in mind what environmental and architectural conditions you're likely to encounter. Say, for example, you're going to France and want to visit several cathedrals in rural villages. In that case, consider renting a wheelchair with wide-track inflatable tires once you arrive, rather than taking along your narrow-tire model. Remember, throughout Europe you'll encounter cobblestone streets and walkways galore.

Those cobblestones may be part of the Old World charm but you won't feel very charmed if you've been bounced over them in a narrow-wheeled American-style wheelchair. European models have smaller-diameter, thicker tires that handle those cobblestones with far less jouncing.

For help with wheelchairs or other assistive devices, write to the Red Cross in the capital city of the country you plan to visit. Some, like the British Red Cross, make wheelchairs and other equipment available for up to eight weeks at no charge (a small donation is always welcomed, though).

Getting in shape for your big adventure

If you haven't ventured forth from hospital or home since your injury or illness, if you haven't used the modes of transportation before that you'll use on your trip, or if you haven't been away from home and its comforts for the length of time you're planning, start a program to get yourself ready for your adventure. Begin taking day trips, then two- and three-day excursions (these are often cheaper if taken weekdays and off season), and finally a more extended safari. The idea is to minimize the number of surprises you're likely to encounter.

These preliminary "shakedown cruises" are often as rewarding as an extended trip. Interesting places lie within fairly easy reach. Chances are you're not too far removed from a metropolitan area, for example. Go for an overnight stay at a center-city hotel. Book a walking tour, eat in an ethnic restaurant, take in the ballet, a concert, browse in a bookstore, or shop in a department store. If you live in a big city, plan an overnight trip to the country. Perhaps you can make a quick trip to the desert or the seashore.

Nearby tourist attractions abound in every state. And, sadly, not many of us who live near them ever take advantage of their proximity. Here's a chance to change that and learn a bit of local lore at the same time. If you live in northern California and enjoy the outdoors, for instance, you might try the Independence Trail outside Nevada City. The trail is actually an ancient flume that once carried water to gold miners, but John Olmsted concluded that it was exactly the right size and pitch (it's five feet wide and drops about ten feet per mile) to become a wheelchair hiking trail. John raised money to extend the two-mile trail through a small group called Sequoya Challenge (P.O. Box 1026, Nevada City, Calif. 95959). The organization is named for the Indian chief who invented an alphabet. ("He was born lame," John notes, "so he, too, was a disabled person.") Roger West has a similar boardwalk in the outdoors not far from Denver. Roger hopes that eventually his trail will extend seven miles to the top of one of the Twin Peaks, a mountain in Pike National Forest. Roger's trail is eight feet wide and is supported by a nonprofit foundation called Wilderness on Wheels, which can be reached in Denver at (303) 988-2212.

Begin in your own backyard, so to speak. If the day is warm, go for a picnic at your neighborhood park, or visit the local natural history museum. Take a spring drive into the desert or mountains to view the wildflowers, or wander through the zoo or along a yacht harbor. Take these excursions for an hour or two at a time. Go slowly at first and lengthen the time of your outings as you gain confidence and strength. An adventure that exhausts you can set you back both physically and psychologically. It's easy to get discouraged when the slightest action is fatiguing, so don't let it happen in the first place.

Dream all you want, but plan ahead

As we noted earlier, dozens of travel guides can give you detailed tips and tricks for travel to almost any part of the world. We have tried to whet your appetite for travel, point out some of the options, and provide some suggestions we've found useful in our travels.

By now it should be clear that planning is of paramount importance for a successful trip. Without it your adventure could turn into one you'd rather not remember. Remember that the whole *raison d' être* of a vacation is to have a pleasant change of pace and to experience a new environment. You aren't going to achieve that if you become physically exhausted, run out of medication, can't find a hotel with an elevator, or discover at a border that you need a visa.

To make reasonably sure all will go well, begin with the list we made and methodically check off the salient items. Nothing is foolproof, but doing your homework tips the odds in your favor. Take the time to dream, to decide, then to plan. If you do these three things, and maintain your sense of humor and your flexibility, you can't go wrong.

Finally...

Above all, be prepared for adventure. It will crop up when you least expect it. At London's Heathrow Airport, signs urge travelers to report suspicious objects. Helynn thought nothing of them until she reached the airport security barrier. Suddenly, uniformed men converged on Helynn and her entourage; one snatched her empty oxygen tank, which was encased in a smart leather bag, and ran.

"That's Aunt Helynn's tank," nephew Larry yelled as he raced after the guard.

Other guards hurried Helynn and her attendant to a less crowded area for questioning.

"They thought we were carrying a bomb," Helynn remembers. "Me! An Irish Republican Army terrorist! My grandmother was Ulster Protestant, for heaven's sake!"

CHAPTER SEVEN

When It's Time to Relax

All of us need some kind of recreation. Our bodies crave the relaxation that results from getting up from behind the desk and going out for a game of basketball, and our minds need a chance to let the stress of daily living wash away. Recreation refreshes us, relaxes us, and lets us return to our tasks with a new perspective.

Sports and other activities

Four wheelchair-bound paraplegic young men crewed aboard a sailboat in the 1988 Los Angeles-Ensenada (Mexico) yacht race. When a television reporter asked one of the men why he was doing it, he replied: "For the adventure." That's reason enough for trying almost anything. It doesn't have to be an international yacht race; for some of us a drive to the countryside can be an adventure. The important thing is to do it. Recreational opportunities for the disabled are everywhere. You usually only have to make a few calls to find out what and where. You name the activity—archery, bowling, marathon-running, golf, bicycling, and

---

Biking

The Hand-Bike is an arm-powered bicycle its manufacturers say offers all the enjoyment of bicycling, even over rough terrain. The bike has a wide gear range, weighs about forty-five pounds, and will cruise at speeds in excess of ten miles an hour. A racing version is also available.

For more information, contact Recreational Mobility, Inc., P.O. Box 147, Elmira, Ore. 97347 (Phone: [503] 935-2828).

---

on and on—and a disabled person somewhere is participating and having a good time. People in wheelchairs continue to square-dance, ice-skate, fly planes, play basketball, shoot the white water in rubber rafts, and ski. Don't just sit at home and watch television. Get out and do something.

Physical activity of some sort helps keep our bodies "in tune," but we don't always jump anxiously to engage in physically strenuous pursuits, even though we know we should. Consider the number of people, disabled or not, who admit they need to exercise but consider it a chore. However, if we can associate physical activity with pleasure in any way, we are more apt to do it regularly.

Going to physical therapy is not nearly as much fun as going swimming, for example. Swimming can be excellent therapy (in fact, many therapists conduct sessions in the water) or simple relaxation. In either case, it can benefit muscular coordination. Helynn grew up on an island in the Susquehanna River in Pennsylvania, and swimming was second nature to all the kids on the island. Besides the river, a large public pool was open all summer long. After becoming a polio quadriplegic at age eight, Helynn continued swimming.

"I had to wear a small air-filled life ring," she remembers. "But being able to go in the water with my friends just as before helped me to remain 'one of the gang' psychologically. When I would drift too far downstream on the river current, one of the kids would just tow me back."

Perhaps a family member or neighbor has a backyard pool. If

so, and if you haven't discovered the pleasures of swimming, dive in some warm day. Because water lessens the effects of gravity, you'll find it is easier to move about on your own. The discovery that you can get from here to there alone is an exciting revelation. (Incidentally, if you're looking for a place to swim, contact your local YMCA, rehabilitation department, or city parks and recreation department for information.)

As far as sports activities are concerned, let us offer one caution: before you charge off to run a marathon or join a wheelchair basketball team (the national association's address is in the appendix), make sure you check with your doctor. Give yourself every opportunity for a rewarding activity, be it running or dancing, by making certain you're in good health before you begin.

Also bear in mind that your recreational activities may be governed to one degree or another by conditions that may be beyond your control. Some things you may want to be involved in may not be within your range of ability, and others may not be available where you live. But even if you can't get as completely involved as you'd like, you can probably participate in the same activity to a lesser extent. Perhaps you won't be able to fly an airplane but still have a passion for aviation. Well, there's model aviation as an alternative, or perhaps you can find a private pilot who'd like to have a navigator along on short trips. Remember, there's always something you can do.

Wheelchair dancing and wheelchair basketball are two of the most familiar activities in which the disabled participate, perhaps because of their visual impact and impressiveness. But sports and leisure activities aren't limited to just those things, as we all know. Disabled individuals have climbed sheer rock faces like Half Dome in Yosemite, hiked rugged mountain trails, and landed some very hefty fish. And the range of disabilities "represented" in these accomplishments is amazing: polio, muscular dystrophy, multiple sclerosis, and cerebral palsy patients; amputees; and those left paraplegic from diving, car, or train accidents.

The point, of course, is that a disability need not end your active leisure life. You don't have to go chasing up a mountainside if that doesn't appeal to you, but some sort of sport-like activity

Exercise Videos

Workout videos are all the rage these days, and several are on the market specifically for the disabled. A phone call to a local fitness center or gym might provide you with more.

An exercise program entitled *Wheelchair Aerobics* features routines for the neck, shoulders, arms, and trunk. The tape also shows how elastic bands made especially for workouts can complement these exercises.

Wheelchair Aerobics stresses exercising within the framework of health and abilities; the exercises can be modified to ensure an appropriate pace. The routines in the half-hour video are performed by individuals with various physical limitations and are led by an aerobics instructor.

For more information about *Wheelchair Aerobics,* contact Cindy Collet Hodges, A/V Health Services, Inc., P.O. Box 20271, Roanoke, Va. 24018 (Phone [703] 772-0659 or [703] 389-5724).

The Michigan Amputee Foundation also has a video of low-impact aerobics designed primarily for amputees. For more information contact Terry Willis, Michigan Amputee Foundation, 6849 So. Division Ave., Grand Rapids, Mich. 49508 (Phone [616] 281-2002).

The New York City chapter of the National Multiple Sclerosis Society sells the *M.S. Workout Video Tape* for fifteen dollars. It

will help keep you fit and mentally alert. Just think of some of the things you can do: dance, play basketball, camp, fish, hunt, hike, ride horses, climb mountains, play tennis, go white-water rafting, run. As we said before, the list is very long.

Once you identify an activity you'd like to try, spend some time familiarizing yourself with it. Check it out with your doctor to make sure you can handle the exertion, then set out to learn about it. If you're interested in something sponsored by a national organization for the disabled, you might contact that group for information. Many such organizations are listed in the appendix of this book. You can usually make contact with organizations in your area through a local sporting goods store that outfits people features Jimmy Heuga, 1964 Olympic skier and founder of a center that promotes physical exercise and fitness for persons with disabilities, along with members of the New York City chapter, in a routine of warm-ups, calisthenics, cool-downs, and relaxation exercises.

To get this tape, contact the New York City chapter, National Multiple Sclerosis Society, 30 West 26th St., 9th Floor, New York, N.Y. 10010.

Fitness Is for Everyone is a series of videotapes available for $14.50 from National Handicapped Sports, 1145 19th St., N.W., Suite 717, Washington, D.C. 20036.

Keep Fit While You Sit is a $29.50 tape sold by Slabo Productions, 1057 So. Crescent Heights Blvd., Los Angeles, Calif. 90035.

Television diet and exercise guru Richard Simmons also has a video for the disabled. It concentrates on strengthening and stretching exercises and is entitled *Reach for Fitness*. It costs $14.98 from Karl-Lorimar Home Video (your local video store can order it for you).

In every case, specify whether you need Beta or VHS format.

In addition, you can get an audio cassette and handbook, *Wheelchair Workout*, for $16.75 from Janet Reed, 12275 Greenleaf Ave., Potomac, Md. 20854 (Maryland residents add appropriate sales tax).

One magazine dealing with sports and fitness is *Sports 'n' Spokes*, published bimonthly by Paralyzed Veterans of America, 5201 No. 19th Ave., Suite 111, Phoenix, Ariz. 85015.

---

for the sport. Ask for the phone number of a club, then ask about others who are disabled and involved in this activity.

Then, before you've committed a tremendous amount of money and time to this activity, make a trial run. Find a disabled acquaintance (able-bodied if you can't find an experienced disabled partner) and make a short run down a river or a short climb. Try it out. How do you like it? Does the experience leave you exhilarated and wanting more? Or are you glad it's over? You'll be able to judge quickly whether or not you want to continue with this particular activity. By the way, many outdoor activities (camping, fishing, and even some hiking) require licenses or permits. Make sure you check local regulations.

Flying

Just because you're in a wheelchair or otherwise limited doesn't mean you have to be cut off from many of the activities life has to offer. Having his wings clipped was a terrible blow to Bill Blackwood. He had always loved flying; he'd received his license at twenty-four, when he joined the Navy. Suddenly, after his plane accident in 1962, he was forty and grounded. For sixteen happy years he'd been a naval aviator. It ended when he had to eject from his aircraft. The accident hospitalized him for a year and left him a paraplegic.

In 1963, convinced he wouldn't be able to go back to flying, he moved to Southern California, where he sold real estate. But the love of flying continued to nag at him.

"For five years after the accident, I was still interested in flying, but I didn't think I could continue," he recalls. "Then I came to the realization that my lack of leg use could be overcome with hand controls.

"Others had flown with hand controls before me. They'd buy their own aircraft and have the controls installed. But I realized that owning a plane was not realistic. So in 1968 I developed a portable hand control that could be adapted to any plane. Other paraplegics who wanted to continue flying heard about it and contacted me. I made them for six or seven years and sold 250 throughout the world. FAA [Federal Aviation Administration] personnel assisted me. We had to have everything checked—the engineering drawings, flight tests—to make sure it worked in flight. Anytime you modify an airplane in any way you have to get FAA approval." Blackwood gave up real estate and went back to flying. In 1972 he received the Flight Instructor of the Year certificate.

Blackwood not only invented portable hand controls for disabled pilots, he also founded the California Wheelchair Aviators (in 1974). It began with only three pilots but now has 128 around the world.

Hobbies

Originally, what we know as the word *hobby* referred to hawking, a pastime of feudal nobility not unlike falconry. Nowadays, we've broadened the term to include things a person likes to do or study in his or her spare time.

"We fly all over the Western states," Blackwood says. The pilots fly somewhere once a month "either for lunch, or to spend two or three days. We pick a spot and fly to it," says Blackwood, whose organization's headquarters are at 1117 Rising Hill Way, Escondido, Calif. 92025 (Phone: [619] 746-5018).

Blackwood points out proudly that a few of the Wheelchair Aviators have even appeared in air shows. "One pilot in our group, who's from Idaho, can do air-show aerobatics," he says. "He had flown a biplane in air shows throughout the U.S. and two years ago was in an accident. Now he's a paraplegic, but he got right back into aerobatics."

Federal regulations governing private pilots are very strict to begin with. Blackwood had to prove that disabled pilots could control an airplane satisfactorily. To be licensed, however, disabled pilots must earn both a certificate of demonstrated ability and a supplemental-type certificate.

Donald (Rodey) Rodewald of Colorado was the second disabled pilot to buy one of Blackwood's portable hand controls and became the first paraplegic to solo around the world. He had been an Army Air Corps pilot and had been in an accident in January 1954 at Andrews Field outside Washington, D.C. That accident left him a paraplegic but did not end his love of flying.

A veteran of the China theater in World War II and a fighter pilot in Korea, Rodewald flew in military air shows before his accident. Once he found that he could use a hand control for the rudder operation, he was off in the air again. "It was easy for me to adapt to the hand control after only three hours' training," he says. In 1984, he flew his single-engine Piper Comanche 31,350 nautical miles around the world. He spent three and a half months and made thirty-four landings in twenty-four countries.

"The battle of government bureaucracies was the most frustrating part," he recalls. "The flying part was easy."

Almost any enjoyable activity can be called a hobby, and sometimes (and not so seldom as you might think) a hobby can become a vocation. Often the income generated by a hobby is not enough to support you, although it can be a welcome supplement to your bank account. People whose job and hobby are the same are generally highly successful. If you generally love what you are

Dancing

The Arizona Square Wheelers started less than ten years ago with eight members. The group performs at various functions in the Phoenix area and has participated with able-bodied dancers in the twenty-four-hour state dance-a-thon to help raise money for the Jerry Lewis Muscular Dystrophy Telethon.

The dancers' motto is "We can't dance on our feet so we dance on our seats." Performer Millie Mislevich says: "We've become very good friends. I think we all care for each other in a very natural way."

The dancers say they generally do all the steps any other square-dance group does, with a few exceptions. The do-si-do, for example, requires three steps sideways, and that's a little difficult on wheels. Caller Jim Strava explains: "We just leave out some sideways steps. In others, by modifying the routine a little, we simulate a sideways step."

Strava, who is not disabled, has stuck by the group since it began: "One day, after doing a demonstration with able-bodied people, I

doing, you can't fail. You're certainly less likely to fall victim to stress.

Everyone needs a diversion of some sort once in a while, if for no other reason than as a road to explore other than one's daily routine. If you're housebound, you can definitely benefit from the intellectual and physical stimulation of a hobby.

Spend some time investigating all kinds of hobbies. One way to do this, if you're able, is to visit county fairs and hobby shows. You'll find times and dates in the newspaper. Or check the Yellow Pages. Call the model railroad, ceramics, or archeology club you're interested in. Ask when their next activity is scheduled. Their members are always delighted to entice a potential newcomer.

The more of this kind of exploring you do, the more interested you are likely to become in something you never expected. One aspect of a hobby is its unexpected appeal. Another is its ability to divert you from everyday matters like work or school. Still another is its ability to stimulate your mind. If it doesn't appeal to invited several handicapped people in the audience to join us. And they really had fun. Afterwards, several parents whose handicapped children had joined in came up to me and said, 'I'm sorry my child was in there. He's messing up your show.' I really felt bad to learn some parents would do that to their children. So, when the opportunity came to get with this group, I took the challenge and it kind of grew on me."

Wheelchair-bound dancers don't need to wait until they're with others in wheelchairs to enjoy dancing. Couples in wheelchairs can weave some remarkably intricate patterns on a dance floor crowded with able-bodied dancers.

Helynn square-danced in her manual (but lightweight) Everest and Jennings wheelchair many years ago. Her able-bodied boyfriend enjoyed square dancing, so off they went.

"He saw no reason why we shouldn't participate," Helynn remembers. "I was the only disabled person on the floor. I am glad to report that this did not appear to bother any of the dancers. They would simply swing my chair in the circle without missing a step or a word of the caller's instructions.

"There's nothing better than a date to go dancing."

you, doesn't take your mind off the day-to-day, and doesn't make you think, you probably won't stay with it very long. When you go to hobby shows, keep these things in mind. Talk to exhibitors and to the people hanging around the displays. If something isn't your cup of tea, fine. You've still learned something new, and that's always to your advantage.

Another excellent way to investigate the hobby scene, again depending on your mobility, is to explore hobby shops in your area. By their very nature they offer a wealth of information, including the costs of pursuing a particular activity. A too-expensive hobby can keep you worried about meeting the bills, which is hardly attractive. A hobby has to be fun, a diversion, and within your means, both financially and physically. If it becomes a burden, it's time to find something else.

It's helpful in your decision-making process to keep a "daydream diary" of hobbies in which you're interested. Separate the activities you've explored into two categories: doables (like wine- and

Fishing

"My father used to take me trout fishing in the Pennsylvania mountains," Helynn remembers. "The beauty of the forest, the bird calls, and the glimpses of squirrels, deer, chipmunks, and the imagined sound of a bear in the thick underbrush sent delicious shivers down my spine.

"I would sit with the wheels of my chair in the stream, a sandwich in my lap, and a trout rod balanced on the arm of the chair—alone in the wilderness. Since you really can't fish for trout unless you wade in the stream, my father with all his gear would disappear for an hour or two at a time.

"Since I never caught a fish on any of our expeditions, it's clear that being alone in the forest was my real reason for going. That and the look of astonishment on the face of an occasional fisherman who, on rounding a bend in the stream, would see a skinny young girl hub-deep in the water eating a chicken sandwich!"

An electric retrieve fishing reel designed for freshwater fishing and powered by 6- or 12-volt rechargeable batteries or a cigarette-lighter power cord is available from Royal Bee Corp. It frees fishermen with physical handicaps of their rod-holding harnesses. The Bee is operated by casting, then retrieving using the push-button electric retrieve. For additional information contact Royal Bee Corporation, 703 Kihekah, Pawhuska, Okla. 64056 (Phone: [918] 287-1044).

For ocean fishing, other automatic retrieve reels are available. Check catalogs listed in the appendix.

beermaking) and collectibles (like stamps and coins). Some, like model-boat building, may fit in both categories. Rate the relative cost for each hobby. Then list the things about each hobby that interest you most. Next, list the things you'd like to do in that activity. You'll have a "cluster" of ideas about and aspects of each hobby. These things add up to the degree of complexity involved in the activity; and some hobbies will, by nature, have greater complexity levels than others. Radio-controlled model airplanes, for instance, can appeal to you from a variety of standpoints: construction, design experimentation, military or civilian time-period modeling, engine tuning and repair, solar power, aerobatic flight, glider flight, and so forth. Kite-flying may possess some of the same elements, but you probably won't have as many in that cluster. The cost of the latter will be significantly lower, though.

Examine each cluster. See what level of complexity appeals to you most. Just remember that, despite your limited physical ability or your uncertain cash flow, you'll find more hobbies than you'll ever find time to give to them. Don't worry about gender distinctions, either. Most hobbies these days attract members of both sexes because of what they have to offer—not because they are specific to one gender or the other.

Thousands of hobbies are waiting to absorb you. You can, for example, collect almost anything: stamps, coins, baseball cards, antique bottles, seashells, rocks, comic books, postcards, or miniatures for a doll's house. You could try short-wave radio broadcasting, model railroading, or winemaking. All such activities challenge us intellectually and so attract and hold our attention.

If you're looking for something to get you out of doors but not too far from home, you might try gardening. A fascinating variety of options exists here, including orchid-growing, indoor gardening, or *bonsai* (Japanese miniature tree culture). Another universally popular hobby is photography, and a variety of specially designed equipment is available for the disabled. Contact Special Needs Adapted Photography, Polaroid Corp., 784 Memorial Dr., Cambridge, Mass. 02139, for detailed product information.

The parks and recreation department

If you haven't already done so, call your city's parks and recreation department and ask to be put on their mailing list. You'll receive their monthly or quarterly activity calendar, and you may find some pleasant surprises from an organization you've overlooked or taken for granted for a long time.

Some cities have special programs for the physically disabled, but many don't. Regardless, don't overlook the department that doesn't have special programs. You're looking for activities that

A Fishing Pole and a Gun Are His Tools
BY LES CARROLL

The cement plant foreman, wearing a hard hat, frowned at the freelance writer who had come to do a story about the new temperature-proof buildings atop one of his towers.

"Oh, I didn't know you were in a wheelchair," he said, embarrassed. "I'm afraid this won't work out."

"Well, let's take a look at it," replied Jack Nelson, writer and college professor, who had driven more than a hundred miles from his Provo, Utah, home to gather information and take photographs. A half hour later, after a noisy ride up the elevator to the top of the 200-foot-high towers, Jack got the story and pictures he needed to complete the assignment he had contracted to write for a large East Coast trade publication.

Getting a job done has never been a problem for Nelson, who has used a wheelchair for thirty-five years. In fact, as an avid outdoorsman, accomplished writer, journalism professor, husband, and father, he probably has more success than most people when it comes to getting the things important to him.

"People are surprised that I'm a hunter, or at least a *successful* hunter," explains Nelson, who bagged his first deer in 1951 and has averaged one a year since then. He adds: "I probably have more patience and better concentration than most hunters, because I've had to learn those assets to be successful."

As a California schoolboy Nelson lettered in football and track. In his final season of track, when a numbness developed in his feet and toes, he broke nine hurdles in one week. A week later he was in the hospital with a condition called transverse myelitis. He had total sensory and motor loss below the seventh thoracic vertebra.

"I remember thinking," Nelson says, "that the worst thing about it all was that I would not be able to hunt or fish anymore, which, as a boy, I loved more than anything."

But in college, he learned he could compete successfully with his

are challenging, fun, and relaxing as well as mentally stimulating. Your parks department with its array of events could be able to supply you with just the thing you're looking for.

Recreation specialist Debra Harvey has worked for the city of roommate cousin—with a fishing pole, a shotgun, or hosting week-end dates.

"We went duck hunting a couple of times a week and had a contest to see who could shoot the most ducks over the season," he says. "We tied, and that incident helped change my attitude. It taught me that I could compete in the things I loved doing, and ever since then I have had no trouble accepting what happened."

Nelson quickly learned that for a hunter, a steady arm and good aim were nearly as good as two strong legs. He also found he could use the patience he had learned to his advantage when hunting or fishing.

"If I can get in a good spot, and if I'm patient and quiet, eventually a deer will come along," Nelson says. "I remember ten years ago going to Colorado to hunt elk and coming home with the only elk in a party of nine hunters."

Jack received a doctorate in journalism from the University of Missouri in 1971. Today the fifty-three-year-old Nelson is an assistant professor of journalism at Brigham Young University. Ten years ago he published his first novel, the story of D.B. Cooper, the first person to hijack an airplane for money. That book, entitled *The Parajacker*, was published under the pseudonym Jeremiah Jack. Two other novels followed. A few years ago Nelson decided to combine his love of the outdoors with his skills as a writer, and he began writing articles for outdoor magazines. He presently does most of his work for *Western Outdoors*, of which he is Utah editor and a feature contributor.

"It's nice when I can grab my gun or fishing equipment and tell my wife I'm going to work," he says. "I have a good time, make a little money, and do what I love to do."

He and his wife Patrice have three children, one of whom is a Navajo boy named Jedediah. "To me, they are not really adopted," says Nelson about his son and two daughters. And to Nelson, he's not really handicapped. As long as his family, his writing, teaching, and the great outdoors are all a part of his life, then he has no handicaps.

San Diego since 1976 and, since 1981, has worked with the disabled. "We have to be aware of the adaptations necessary to help the disabled get the most out of their recreation activities," she says, reflecting something you'll find among most recreation

Recreation Publications

A disabled recreation newspaper...

Disabled Outdoors is a quarterly newspaper designed to inform disabled sportspersons about a wide variety of outdoor activities. The newsletter is a clearinghouse for specialized information and new products as well as a source of encouragement to sportspersons with disabilities who want to get involved in outdoor activities.

For more information, contact *Disabled Outdoors*, 5223 So. Lorel Ave., Chicago, Ill. 60638.

... And outdoor catalogs

Access to Recreation, Inc., has a catalog of adaptive recreation equipment that features more than a hundred items, ranging from a ten-dollar Quad-Bee, a frisbee for quadriplegics, to a six-thousand-dollar all-terrain amphibious vehicle with hand controls.

For this catalog, write Access to Recreation, 2509 E. Thousand Oaks Blvd., Suite 430, Thousand Oaks, Calif. 91360 (Phone: 1-800-634-4351; in California [805] 498-7535).

Stuart's Sports Specialties is another catalog that includes a variety of sports items for people with disabilities. The publication was developed by Stuart Reder of Alaska following a 1983 motorcycle accident that left him partly paralyzed. It represents the results of Reder's search for equipment to facilitate his pursuit of sports activities. Most items in the catalog have been tested for quality. Merchandise includes a carbine for one-handed shooting, a hand-loading press, a fishing harness, a one-handed pocket survival tool, and an automatic boat loader. The catalog costs a dollar. To order, contact Stuart's Sport Specialties, 7081 Chad St., Anchorage, Alaska 99502 (Phone: [907] 349-8377).

Those who enjoy fishing, hunting, camping, or other outdoor activities can find specially designed equipment in J.L. Pachner's *Products to Assist the Disabled Sportsman* catalog. It's free and lists (with photos) dozens of useful items. Write J.L. Pachner, Ltd., 33012 Lighthouse Court, San Juan Capistrano, Calif. 92675.

specialists—an acute awareness of disabled needs. "We take the disabled in wheelchairs ice skating—we've had no problem with insurance and the people who operate the ice-skating rink have

More Publications

Numerous organizations provide informational pamphlets and other publications. Here are several dealing with a range of recreational activities for the disabled. To find out about other similar publications, start by contacting the national organization that deals with your disability. Magazines like Accent on Living, Together, Rehabilitation Gazette, *and others often have pertinent information, too.*

"Camping in the National Park System" is available from the Superintendent of Documents, U.S. Government Printing Office, Washington, D.C. 20402, for $3.50. It identifies approximately fifty parks that the National Park Service has cited that have wheelchair-accessible or usable campgrounds.

"Waterskiing for the Physically Disabled" is free from Kathy Wilkinson, c/o Mission Bay Aquatic Center, 1001 Santa Clara Point, San Diego, Calif. 92109 (Phone: [619] 488-1036). This handbook includes recommendations on equipment and techniques based upon the experience of the Mission Bay Aquatic Center ski instructors and staff. Topics include fitness to ski, safety, equipment, starting and skiing, and skier's signals.

Eight manuals are available from Vinland National Center for $6.50 each. Five of the eight are "Pulk Skiing and Ice Sledding for Persons with Mobility Impairments," "Fitness Courses with Adaptations for Persons with Disabilities," "Cross Country Skiing for Persons with Disabilities," "An Introduction to Kayaking for Persons with Disabilities," and "Horseback Riding for Persons with Disabilities." Order from Vinland National Center, Lake Independence, Loretto, Minn. 55357; (Phone: [612] 479-3555).

"Equipment for the Disabled: Leisure and Gardening" edited by E.R. Wilshere and G.M. Cochrane in 1983 has a section on gardening with tips on setting up an accessible greenhouse, pruning trees, and laying out an accessible and easy-upkeep patio garden. Photographs are included and equipment that is available for export overseas is noted. Write the Oxfordshire Health Authority, Noffield Orthopedic Center, Oxford OX3 7LD, Great Britain.

always been cooperative. And we have a bowling league. We have the same type of recreation and leisure activities as everyone else. We have volunteers when we need help with the wheelchairs. We get volunteers from our volunteer coordinator, the United Way, school groups, public service announcements, universities, and other places.

The San Diego parks board issues a monthly newsletter listing activities especially for the disabled. Check with your own parks department and participate in some events. You'll widen your circle of friends and add zest to your everyday life.

Do it for the fun of it

We haven't even begun to scratch the surface of the things you can do, but we can't stress too much the importance of finding *something* to do. Every one of us needs an activity or two to relieve the stress of making a living and take our minds off our worries. Recreational and hobby activities serve that purpose. Whether building model airplanes or boats, casting and painting toy soldiers, or writing programs for computer games, if it relaxes and refreshes you, it's worth the time and energy.

CHAPTER EIGHT

Feel Good, Look Better

Your health, your appearance, and your life-style are all woven together. This chapter deals with the first two; life-style is what the rest of this book is about. Our message is a simple one: don't underestimate the importance of health and appearance. To a great extent, your life-style depends on your health; in some ways—job hunting, for instance—your life-style can depend on appearance, too. Be careful not to fall victim to the notion that because of your disability you are somehow exempt by a compassionate society from making an effort to be healthy and to look and feel attractive.

Remember: your outward appearance reveals a lot about your physical *and* emotional health. The inner glow of a healthy person is an attractive magnet that draws everyone's admiring attention. That look of health *is* beauty; those of us who don't have it must work diligently to achieve it.

Meanwhile, we need to maintain good grooming habits and choose clothing to fit both our bodies and our personalities. Taking an interest in how you look is a giant step toward both physical and emotional health—for men as well as women.

Health

Health isn't something you can fake or produce by sleight-of-hand, as you can some other things. Your health must come first or you will feel too miserable to do much of anything. Contrary to the attitude held by some, good health—basic, straightforward good health—can be achieved by the disabled. You may be physically disabled, but that doesn't mean you have to lie in bed day after day being sickly. In fact, the maintenance of your overall health will minimize the negative drain on your energy caused by your specific disability.

You can take steps right now, today, to be a healthy person. First, commit yourself to constant attention to your health and to improving your health. The importance of this idea cannot be stressed enough. You can do several things to keep yourself in condition and in good health in spite of your disability. The specifics of these things will vary from disability to disability, but the same principles of good health still apply.

How can anyone walk unscathed through the minefields of health services? Very carefully! If you take the time to reflect on what you are doing to your body during your daily activities, you should find yourself in a position where you know enough to exercise some common sense about how to care for yourself in a positive way. Unless you learn all you can about the things that affect your health, you won't be able to make the sound decisions essential to improve your health and to maintain your continued well-being. In other words, make the decision to take charge of your health with the same resolve with which you tackled school, job hunting, and travel.

Although your health should be taken seriously, try to be just a bit light-hearted as you approach the task. After all, good health is a life-long pursuit. Enjoy it.

The following categories all contribute to improving or maintaining your health:

- Following medical advice
- Medication
- Nutrition

- ♦ Exercise
- ♦ Rest
- ♦ Teeth
- ♦ Skin

Regular attention to these basic health factors can help improve your general health.

Following medical advice

If there's one bit of tried and true advice that's more important than anything else we could suggest about health, it's this: pay attention to what your doctor tells you. Your doctor will provide you a road map to health; follow it. You'll feel good and look good.

Following the doctor's advice is viewed differently by the patient, the caregiver, and the family and friends of the patient. One caution: only you and your doctor can devise a routine—for exercise or anything else—that feels comfortable and that produces the results you want. An overly ambitious plan won't succeed because you probably won't stick to it. Sooner or later, we all learn that. How many people do you know who have tried restrictive weight-loss programs? One of two things usually happens: either they give up after a few days or they eventually gain back the weight they lost and more. A health routine is like a diet: if you place too many unrealistic demands on yourself, you're not likely to succeed. It's best to start any new course of action slowly, one step at a time. Whatever you do, go about it sensibly and do it in moderation. That way you're more likely to stick to it.

Medication

Gather together all the medicines you take on a daily or occasional basis. Put them all on your bed table or desk. Does the quantity surprise you? More important, have you discussed them all with your doctor? The fact is that often over-the-counter nonprescription drugs and drugs prescribed by your doctor do not mix. But in our quest to get well or feel better, we seldom think of that.

Now that you have taken a long look at what's in your personal pharmacy, list all the drugs. Start with those prescribed by your doctor, then add those over-the-counter medicines you bought at the local drugstore. Record the doctor's name and the dosage for each prescription, followed by what you are taking it for. For over-the-counter drugs, record the dosage and the reason you are taking them. Now you have a straightforward record of the medicines you are taking and—undoubtedly—a much clearer picture of what you are putting into your body.

On your next visit, take the list with you and discuss it with your doctor. Ask the following questions:

♦ What is it for?
♦ What does it do?
♦ What are the side effects?
♦ How will it react with my other medicines?

Keep your list up to date so that you have a handy and accurate reference for you and your doctor to consult. You can't expect your doctor to remember all your medication, especially if you have more than one physician. Also, you can't expect him or her to know what you pick up on your own at the drugstore. Your doctor needs to know *all* the medications you take because many drugs are counterproductive when taken together and some combinations are actually lethal.

Common sense should also remind you to monitor your reactions to all medications and report them to your primary physician. Don't wait a week or two in hopes that the nausea or the ringing in your ears will subside. You gain no points for enduring discomfort, and some reactions can be life-threatening. Something as simple as nose drops can turn into a nightmare of swollen membranes, bleeding, sinus infections, and loss of sense of smell that takes a doctor to clear up. Read the label. Never take any medicines longer than the directions advise and never increase the dosage.

Many medications are addictive, so caution in taking prescription drugs is a must. You can't very well take charge of your life if chemicals are controlling your emotions. If you have a temporary need for mood-altering medication, be sure to use it only temporarily.

Periodically check the medicine's expiration date and promptly discard all those that are outdated. Throwing away an old prescription is not extravagant, no matter how much it may have cost in the first place. Medicine can lose its potency with age or become dangerous because of changes it undergoes with the passage of time. When it comes to medicine, play it safe.

If you want to learn about the various side effects of different medicines, you can pick up one of the several books that list medicines by both trade and generic names. The best known is the *Physician's Desk Reference*. Most will identify the illnesses the medicine was developed to combat and all known side effects. Such books are inexpensive and useful to have on hand.

Nutrition

Nutrition is an aspect of living that is vital if we're going to be consistently healthy. We don't have to count calories or swear off favorite desserts, but we need to make sure we eat the right kinds of foods. This is especially true for someone who's disabled, and especially for someone who's confined to bed or a wheelchair. Dozens of excellent books on nutrition are available; get one and read it. Learn what foods your body needs, and make sure you include them in your diet. Check with your doctor, too, about whether it's okay to take vitamins and minerals as a dietary supplement. Chances are you can, but it pays to be sure.

If you are confined to bed or to a wheelchair, you may have to pay closer attention to your weight than you would if you were able-bodied and active. And, from time to time, you might find your weight creeping up beyond acceptable limits. Put away all those crash diet books and take a sensible look at yourself and your eating habits. If you do this, you can generally come up with a perfectly satisfactory answer to your eating problem. In the first place, few people really have any "eating problems" other than overindulgence in snack foods while watching TV. If that's the case with you, just knock off the fried, iced, or sugared stuff.

There are physiological reasons why some people persist in

being over- or underweight, no matter how much, how little, or what they eat. Sometimes one's metabolism or glands run amok. If you suspect this might be the case with you, talk to your doctor. Most important, follow his or her advice. Don't try to cure yourself. These malfunctions can seriously threaten your overall health.

Another thing you may need to check if you are having eating problems is whether you have any food allergies. Very few people have a glandular or metabolic problem; a great many have one or more allergies. Milk products, wheat, eggs, and chocolate are the most common culprits. The best way to find out what you may be allergic to is to see an allergist for a series of tests. The tests are simple to administer and quickly done. Besides foods, allergies can be caused by animals, dust, flowers, anything drifting in your environment.

It is not within the scope of this book to give dietetic advice except to emphasize the importance of good nutrition. And, before you make any drastic changes in your diet, make sure you check with your doctor.

Exercise

Okay, so you don't want to pump iron. No one is going to insist or even suggest you become Mr. or Ms. Universe. Aside from that, what do you really have against exercise? Whatever your prejudice against exercise might be, shelve it for a while and make up your mind to give it a try.

The first thing you ought to do is find out from your doctor and physiotherapist what you should be doing to counter the effects of your particular disability. This is the most important step in setting up your exercise regimen. The wrong kind of exercise and overexercise can be harmful rather than helpful. Set up a program that will benefit you and be enjoyable at the same time. Once it has been determined what you need to be doing to strengthen your muscles, look at alternative sorts of things you can also do, things like isometrics, yoga, and aerobics. All of these can be modified so that you can do them to a helpful degree no matter how disabled you are.

If you can get out to exercise classes, that is the best way to go. When you set a time to attend regular classes, you are more apt to stick to it. For leads to supplemental activities of this sort, check with your local parks and recreation department, the nearest YMCA or YWCA, or nearby recreation centers. Refer to Chapter 7 for suggestions about these subjects. Even though you may not fall into the age group, call senior citizen organizations in your area and inquire about swimming and other kinds of exercise classes. They are aimed toward the less strenuous routines.

Some private health clubs and spas have also developed specialized classes for the disabled. Call one and ask what they have in your city. Many have produced videotapes. Check with a video store to learn what might be available. The market in exercise tapes changes quickly, so if you don't find what you want this week call back in a month. Search until you find a tape you can comfortably follow. Chapter 7 also lists information about aerobics videos specifically for the disabled.

The easiest form of exercise is done in a warm-water pool. The water's natural buoyancy lessens somewhat the pull of gravity and gives you a freedom of movement not possible on land. In this gentle floating environment, you can exercise your muscles for a longer time before you begin to tire. If you can't swim, have an attendant or a friend help you. When you go through your exercise routine you need someone to help even if you can swim. Have the friend hold your head above the water while you go through the routine. Do the same here as you would out of water. Notice how much easier it is and how much you can do before you tire.

On a par with swimming, yoga can be an equally easy and helpful form of exercise. But before you buy books and attempt it yourself, look for a teacher who has some knowledge of physical disabilities, one who will be able to adapt the yoga method to your particular capabilities. Yoga is an age-old form of exercise and muscle training that builds a healthy body—and many aspects of yoga can be of paramount importance in maintaining the muscle tone and general health of every disabled person. No one is so physically disabled that he or she cannot do some of the

Sleep Disorders

Many serious sleep disorders are collected under the umbrella term *sleep apnea*. If you suspect that you might suffer from more than simple occasional insomnia, talk to your doctor. Most sleep disorders can be effectively treated once they have been accurately diagnosed.

Your doctor might send you to a sleep disorder clinic. This clinic will be staffed by technicians and doctors who are trained in the field of sleep-related problems: psychologists, neurologists, and pulmonary specialists all working together to solve your dilemma.

The primary symptoms of sleep disorders include periods of anxiety, a constant state of depression, breathing problems (especially during the night hours), abnormal leg movements such as involuntary muscle twitching, and the long-term use of sleep medication. Sleep disorders and these symptoms can have an adverse effect on your other physical disabilities. Among the ill effects of sleep apnea are daytime fatigue, cardiac abnormalities, high blood pressure, and changes in personality.

suggested practices. Celestial Arts in Berkeley, California, has published a book called *Gentle Yoga* with a section geared to the disabled.

Calisthenics are exercises we all remember from our schooldays. If you are still in school, talk to your gym teacher, who will probably be happy to teach you those parts of the calisthenics regimen you can do even if you are in a wheelchair. If you're out of school, phone the physical education department and find a teacher who would come to your house for a few times to get you started in the right direction. But check with your doctor or physiotherapist first to make sure you can handle the exertion and the high-impact nature of calisthenics.

Exercises are like diets: we each have our own built-in prejudices. Besides, the fads in both change rapidly, so ignore the fad of the day and do what feels good. Your body will tell you if you have embarked on the proper set of exercises or not. You should feel tired afterward, but you should also feel invigorated, refreshed, and relaxed.

Going to a sleep clinic is stepping into a futuristic environment. First, your symptoms are identified. Then you're escorted to a small, pleasant room with a comfortable bed. After you lie down, a network of wires is fastened to your arms, chest, and legs. Wires are attached to several places on your head. By this time, if you are alert, you notice the one-way window in the wall. Through it, the doctors, psychologists, and technicians can watch you sleep. (As if all those wires running to banks of equipment in the room beyond the window weren't enough!) After the wires are all connected, someone says "Go to sleep." Suddenly, you're alone in the dark.

Sleep! All tied up and attached to machines that record muscle movement, brainwaves, heartbeat, respiration, and heaven knows what else. Fortunately, all this equipment is in another room, so you don't hear the hums and buzzes or see the iridescent green computer lines zigzag, wave, peak, and curve.

You do manage to sleep, somehow, and the next day all the data from the various charts and graphs are collected and analyzed. The final results take several days to collate and correlate but in the end, you and your doctor have a good idea why your sleep is disturbed.

Rest

Rest may seem an odd topic to include under the heading of health, but it is a vital element in our well-being. Rest is simply quiet relaxation. Obviously, rest is important after periods of physical exertion. Rest is also vital to relieve the emotional stress we all encounter every day. The important thing to remember is that we can't drive ourselves mercilessly and without periodic rest, although the temptation to do so may be strong.

You should feel rested and refreshed when you wake up in the morning. If you don't start the day feeling full of energy, no matter what methods of relaxation you use, you'll never quite reach your energy peak. Get a head start on the day's activities with a good night's sleep.

Our individual body rhythms set how much sleep we need every day. The standard eight-hour daily minimum is the average, but that doesn't mean you have to adjust to it. Your sleep needs will vary according to your physical and mental activity levels, as well as your body's physiological needs. Leaving aside the requirements for individuals with sleep disorders, you should be able to easily ascertain your own nightly needs to wake up refreshed and eager to begin a new day. Once you've determined that, make sure you get that amount of sleep every day. If you consistently wake up feeling tired and sluggish, see your doctor right away.

Teeth

Smile at your reflection in the mirror. Do you like what you see? A smile can lighten up your whole day. If it looks good, that is. You have to be just as ruthlessly objective about your smile as you were about your body or your face.

A twinge of pain in a tooth when sipping a cold or hot liquid is something we tend to ignore—and we shouldn't. Too often we tell ourselves "I know I need to go to the dentist, but I'm too busy right now." We need to *find* time. Doctors and dentists alike will tell you that a number of physical disorders can be traced to dental problems. The message is clear: keep your teeth in top shape; don't take them for granted.

The first order of business is to keep your teeth clean. A regular routine of dental hygiene can work wonders, but you have to remember the regular part. Daily brushing, as we have all heard before, is essential for healthy teeth.

Some people may be unable to brush their teeth because of disability or for some other reason. People who can't can instead rinse with carbamide peroxide, which is sold over the counter, usually under the brand name Gly-Oxide. Carbamide peroxide is a gentle foaming antiseptic cleaner specifically for dental hygiene. Use is simple. According to the label: "When normal oral hygiene is inadequate or impossible . . . swish 10 or more drops vigorously after meals." In addition to providing dental hygiene for people whose disability prevents them from brushing, carbamide peroxide might be useful to have along on camping trips or in other circumstances when regular dental hygiene practices aren't practical.

Nor is there any reason these days for anyone to endure crooked, protruding, or unsightly teeth. Nowadays, people of all ages have their teeth aligned using cleverly concealed orthodontics (braces) that are practically invisible. Gone are the unsightly metal contraptions kids had to endure for years. The advancements in this technology, as in the rest of dentistry, have been truly phenomenal. True, corrective dental work is expensive, but many insurance plans cover all or part of the work. (Dental surgery to correct bite malfunction or jaw deformities is almost always covered by insurance.)

You have enough to contend with in life without putting up with dental problems, too. Make sure you keep those twice-yearly visits to the dentist on your calendar. That way you won't see any disappointment when you smile at yourself in the mirror.

Skin

We pay very little attention to our skin until it irritates us. For the disabled—especially those who wear braces and prosthetics—that irritation can come in the form of *decubiti*, or pressure sores. This breakdown of the skin's cells brought about by pressure or rubbing can be the most serious skin problem you'll ever encounter. Pressure sores develop when there is constant pressure on a part of the body over a period of time. The time period varies from person to person. These sores are most apt to appear on the buttocks of a person who sits in a wheelchair all day or on the heels, elbows, or hip bones of someone who is in bed most of the time.

These areas should be examined daily for any sign of red marks on the skin. These are the warning signs of impending pressure sores. Heed these warning signs immediately. Get a doctor's advice and follow it to the letter. Part of that advice will probably include some kind of pad. Air-filled cushions or pads are rapidly being supplanted by the newer water-filled ones, a sort of spinoff from the popular water bed. These are excellent for people in wheelchairs who sit up for long periods of time. For the bed patient, the best thing to use is sheepskin. However, it is difficult to find; you'll probably have to substitute one made of acrylic.

Like any other part of the body, skin requires at least a minimum of care. And, like anything else, when a problem develops that you can't readily correct, get a doctor's advice and follow it exactly.

Appearance

A shampoo company said it best: "You never get a second chance to make a good first impression." No matter what continent or culture, right or wrong, people are judged by how they look. We make a constant series of judgments based on appearance at social gatherings and in the workplace every day. For a disabled person, pursuit of a career and social interaction are difficult enough. There's no sense making things more difficult by ignoring appearance.

It's easy to "let yourself go" when you feel down or depressed. Guard against that. When you give the impression that you don't care how you look, you broadcast a strong negative attitude to the world, and you are showing whoever comes in contact with you that they aren't important enough for you to make the effort to present yourself at your best. You can greet the world with a smile or a frown; you can "dress for success" or you can "dress for failure." Remember that you have to sell yourself not only to a prospective employer but also to people you deal with in every other aspect of your life.

If you're ever in doubt about how to improve your looks, ask an expert. It's well worth the money. Think of it as an investment. For starters, don't look through the pages of the magazines in search of who or what you want to look like. That won't work. Strive instead to enhance your own particular glow, your own beauty that belongs to you and to no one else.

Like it or not, appearance is a very important part of our image. You can create an image that enhances your true self. You are one of a kind, as different from everyone else as a snowflake is different from every other snowflake. Let your uniqueness be the basis upon which you build the image you want to show the world.

Cosmetic prosthetics are becoming more and more common as an alternative to cosmetic surgery. The remarkably realistic devices can be used when, for example, reconstructive surgery isn't possible because of age or for other medical reasons.

According to *People* magazine, about two hundred specialists in cosmetic prosthetics exist in the United States. Among them, the magazine says, is Denis Lee, who works out of the University of Michigan medical school. The prosthetics can be put on in the morning and removed at night, and the cost is surprisingly low: about $1,300 for an ear and $2,000 for an eye or a foot, *People* says.

To learn more about this "medical sculpture" or about specialists in the field, contact a local cosmetic surgeon or a burn center.

Dress for success

How you dress is important: your attire makes a clear social statement about how you feel about yourself. Your wardrobe can reveal things about your political views, too, or your attitude. What you wear, then, becomes an expression of you and your opinion of yourself and your abilities. Be proud of those things and capitalize on them.

Consciously or unconsciously, our wardrobe reflects the kind of person we are. Are you casual? A perfectionist? Or do you prefer quiet understatement? The clothes we choose reflect these attitudes. We also choose clothes to identify what we do. Blue jeans, for example, seem to be consistently in vogue for college students, while conservative suits are generally *de rigueur* for bankers and lawyers.

When choosing clothes, ask yourself a few pertinent questions:

- Does the outfit minimize your disability? (More on this in a moment.)
- Is the garment comfortable? (Can you move or is it too constrictive?)
- Does it work with whatever devices you use to get around?
- Is it durable?
- Is it really "you"? In your mind's eye, how do you look in it? Does it portray your vision of yourself?

These questions are valid for men or women of any age. Just because a lot of people dress badly doesn't mean you have to be one of them. Take a bit of time when you add to your wardrobe and see how the new item will fit in with what you already have.

Which brings us to an important point for consideration: make periodic checks of your closet before you add to what you have. Do it about twice a year. It's a great time to get rid of what you no longer wear to make room for all the new things. If you haven't worn an article of clothing in the past two years, chances are you aren't going to wear it again. If you're young and have outgrown something, give it to someone younger. One of the worst reasons for saving old clothes is the argument, "As soon as I lose a little weight, they will fit again." They've been hanging around while you were gaining the weight; by the time you lose it, everything will be out of style and you won't want to wear it anyway.

Dressing to minimize deformity

A large number of disabling illnesses leave various observable physical deformities in their wake as the illnesses progress. No clothes or cover-up will really eliminate a physical deformity, of course, but a bit of creativity can successfully minimize it.

In Helynn's case, for example, polio left her too thin and with a dropped left shoulder because of a spinal curvature. To minimize these defects she did several things:

◆ Her mother, a dressmaker, put a pad in the left shoulder of all her dresses and blouses.
◆ To show off her tiny waist, Helynn has always worn brightly-colored, wide belts.
◆ To conceal her thinness, she wears blouses with long, full sleeves and full skirts.

These simple little things worked together to "eliminate the negative and accentuate the positive" in Helynn's appearance.

Few of us ever think we look good in front of a mirror, but no matter how badly affected our bodies may be by our particular disabilities, we can still do *something* to emphasize our good points. In order to be able to take stock of your assets and liabilities you should acquire a full-length mirror. Such a mirror can be especially important in a disabled child's home. No matter what the child's gender or disability, children have a burning desire to look and dress like their peers. It's up to parents, of course, to help make this need for conformity at least a partially realizable goal for their child.

But back to you. Now that you have your mirror, stand or sit in front of it dressed as you normally would be. Write down what you see. List the things you like and the things you don't like. It won't be easy. Be fair. We have a built-in concept of what we want to look like that clouds our vision. Very few people are satisfied with the way their bodies look: their hair is the wrong color or graying too fast, they are too short or too tall or too heavy or too thin, their hips or stomach too big . . . the list can be depressingly long. Add to that the litany of a short leg, a bent spine, palsied arms and you've got a real challenge to deal with. Before you can begin the Great Transformation, you have to separate what you *want* to see from what is *actually* there. After that, you can begin the job of creating a new, healthy, and beautiful you.

Sometimes it takes a magician's sleight-of-hand to make a particular deformity seem to disappear. Maybe sometimes it will seem that you're not magician enough. Experiment! Design, color, and fabric all contrive to make you look different. Experiment with the cut of your clothes and with colors that highlight your hair and skin tones. Along the way, don't fall into the "muumuu trap." Overweight people wear these loose-fitting, bright-colored Hawaiian gowns thinking they conceal the fat. They don't. It's okay to wear something comfortable, but don't think you have to hide inside a tent.

Magazines and newsletters devoted to the needs of the disabled are excellent sources for where to buy specialized articles of clothing as well as other personalized intimate apparel. Sears, Roebuck is one company with a well-illustrated catalog of interest to the disabled. Their clothes are fashionable and well-tailored as well as designed for easy dressing. There is a judicious use of such things as velcro closures and the like. The catalog also carries items such as beds, commodes, lifts, and wheelchairs. You should be able to get a copy at any Sears store. If your local store doesn't happen to have one on hand, they'll gladly send one to you.

Grooming

It really doesn't matter how you dress if you don't practice good grooming habits. There simply isn't much you can do with your hair if it hasn't had a shampoo in a week. Cleanliness is equally important to everyone—young, old, male, or female makes no difference. A bit of "spit and polish" will go a long way toward making you look better *and* feel better. Good grooming is absolutely essential, whether you are hunting for a job or a lover.

Grooming begins from a sense of pride, but it also arises out of a need to feel good. A well-groomed person not only looks better; he or she *feels* better. You owe it to yourself, your friends, and your caregivers to insist on a regimen of good grooming for yourself and your attendant as much as you have a right to insist on the cleanliness of your surroundings.

Laziness is one excuse for being unkempt, but it is not an acceptable reason. No matter how tired you think you are or how unnecessary you think it may be, you still need to summon the effort every morning to bathe, brush, comb, shave, or whatnot. There's a routine of preparation in all that which is valuable, and there's an indication of self-respect as well.

That issue of low self-esteem is probably the underlying reason why some people neglect themselves.

"Creating a pleasing appearance is too much trouble," they argue.

"What does it matter how I look?" they ask themselves.

"I can't get out of bed, can't go to school, can't get a job," they intone.

Hold on! Who says you can't? You're the only one making the decision to take control of your life. If you let your low self-esteem take charge, all the self-deprecating prophecies will come true. Make the effort to blend in and it will prove itself worthwhile. Of course, you're different. Of course, there are things you can't do. There are things you can do that other people can't, too. Have enough pride in yourself to take care of yourself, and doors will start to open for you. Remember: any goal worth achieving requires some effort. If it's worth it to you, it's worth working to get.

CHAPTER NINE

There Are Laws, and Then There Are Laws

We have one final and very important bit of advice: get to know your state senator and your state representative *very* well. They will have or be able to find out the answers to many questions concerning laws and regulations in your state.

Every state has its own set of laws concerning the disabled, and we couldn't possibly attempt to summarize them here. They are too different, too varied. For example, you might not know that disabled persons don't have to pay sales tax when they buy a car in Massachusetts. California collects sales tax from the disabled. What about your state? In some states, a car with a "disabled person" license plate cannot be towed if it's in violation of some parking ordinance. The car might contain some item a disabled person needs to stay alive. In other states, the thought that towing a car could be life-threatening hasn't occurred to lawmakers and so cars with "disabled" plates are towed from time to time.

Enter your state senator or state representative. When you're

The Paper Chase

Sadly, *swiftness* and *the bureaucratic process* are contradictory terms. But it would be wonderful if we could rely on government bureaucracies to act swiftly, especially when the disabled must sometimes depend on fast action simply to live.

To say it is demoralizing for a physically helpless person to be at the mercy of a system of questionable competence and with dozens of built-in twists and turns anyway is to drastically understate the case. Helynn's problems, for example, began in July 1988, when her mother died. That death triggered the diversion of both her deceased parents' civil service pensions to her. This brought federal, state, and local agencies together and embroiled Helynn in a snafu as big as the lead character of Franz Kafka's novel *K* experienced. K spent all of his adult life in government buildings, filling out forms without ever being told why.

In the first three months, Helynn had to mail six copies of death certificates from the state to the federal government. Despite this, her mother's pension checks continued to be deposited in the bank—for a full year. Each check had to be returned eventually.

Finally, a year after her mother's death, Helynn was notified by the federal government that she would receive $138 a month from her father's pension and $256 a month from her mother's.

not sure of the laws in your state for some specific aspect of disabled rights, the quickest way to find the answer is to call one of these people. You can call hospitals, state agencies, police precincts, and any number of other places that *should* know the answer but don't. Save the headaches: look up the senator or representative in your phone book.

Both senators and representatives normally maintain offices in their home cities while they're at the state capitol. A small staff will regularly relay requests and information to the politician's office staff at the capitol. And, even though we may think the things we ask about never find their way to the elected official, they do—with regularity.

Helynn confidently (and mistakenly) assumed these checks would arrive, as stated in the notification, on the first of each month. She promptly reported it, as required by law, to her local caseworker.

As a result, her local checks were stopped.

The new ones never arrived.

A blitz of phone calls and letters only complicated things further. Within a five-week period she was notified that: first, her aid had been eliminated (Helynn is a quadriplegic who spends sixteen hours a day in an iron lung); second, her aid had been restored; third, her PCA's salary was being cut $298; fourth, her own check would be cut to $126; and fifth, she had qualified for a ten-cent increase the next month.

This has taken more than two years to resolve. The only way out of the nightmare was through a maze of phone calls, letters, and, on the rare occasions possible, in-person visits to the offices involved.

The way to solve such problems is to identify each person and agency involved and work through the maze as quickly as possible. Meanwhile, especially in a situation like this, keep your U.S. senator or representative as well as their state counterparts completely informed, by frequent letters if possible.

Finally, if the bureaucracy buries even your senator, contact a local television or newspaper reporter and phone the local legal aid organization. Such a story makes great copy, and the public outrage it's sure to generate may help short-cut some twists and turns in the maze.

When you call your senator or representative (and this holds true for U.S. senators and representatives, too), make sure you begin the conversation this way: "Hello. My name is ———, and I'm one of Senator Jones's disabled constituents. I have a question. Can you please...?" The key words are your name, the words *disabled constituent*, and *please*. Each one means something to the person—most often an aide—at the other end of the line. To a politician, *constituent* means "vote." *Disabled constituent* may mean "influential voting bloc." *Please*, of course, signals that you're not trying to set up a confrontation.

As long as you're straightforward and clear in your request for information, you can expect a quick answer. You might even get an answer like the one Gary received some years ago: "We're sorry. We can't answer your question. We should be able to, but the people who should know don't. The senator is asking for an immediate investigation."

The political pecking order is an interesting thing. You let the senator know that you're a voter in his or her district. The senator takes that information to heart and has the staff identify the agency that should have the answer to your question. As a rule, the agency will respond as quickly as possible to the senator, because the senator will vote on funding for that office sooner or later.

After a few calls to your senator's or representative's office, you'll be on a first-name basis with the aide who works there. You'll probably also be on the politician's Christmas-card list. But you'll have something more important: answers to important questions. Any time you can't readily find the answer to something when you can reasonably expect to find a law governing the situation, call your elected officials. That's what your taxes pay them for.

The Americans with Disabilities Act

On July 13, 1990, the Senate passed a bill that was considered to be the most sweeping anti-discrimination measure since the Civil Rights Act of 1964: the Americans with Disabilities Act.

By the end of August 1990, all new buses, trains, and subway cars had to be accessible to people in wheelchairs, and any public mass transportation system had to provide alternate transportation to people unable to board buses or subways. Also, any new or renovated hotels, retail stores, and restaurants had to include accessibility for wheelchairs, and any existing barriers had to be removed, if "readily achievable." The legislation also said that no commercial establishment could deny service to anyone with a disability.

Within two years, all businesses with more than twenty-five employees will be required to change their facilities to accommodate disabled employees, unless they can demonstrate that the

Social Security

Have a problem with your Social Security check or anything having to do with it? You may want to get in touch with the National Organization of Social Security Claimants' Representatives. Their toll-free number is 1-800-431-2804.

The organization will provide you the names and addresses of attorneys in your area who specialize in claims against the Social Security Administration. Most member attorneys work on contingency basis; that is, they get nothing until your case is satisfactorily settled.

required changes would be too costly, too disruptive, or would substantially alter the way they do business. Within three years, telephone companies will have to provide relay services, allowing hearing- and voice-impaired people who have special telephones to place and receive calls from ordinary phones. Also, "key" subway and train stations must be made accessible to the disabled. And, finally, at the end of five years, all trains and subways must have at least one car that is accessible.

The legislation defines a disability as a condition that "substantially limits" a "major life activity," such as walking or seeing, and includes not only those with physical disabilities, but also drug abusers, alcoholics, and people infected with AIDS.

After overcoming several snags that stalled the bill for months, the House approved the final version by a 377 to 28 vote. Senate passage came on a 91 to 6 vote, and President Bush signed the bill into law soon after. The Americans with Disabilities Act promises to be, as Senator Edward M. Kennedy, one of the bill's fifty-nine sponsors, called it, "an emancipation proclamation for the disabled."

We've pretty well touched on most factors in the preceding pages and hope we've given you an overview of the possibilities available for benefiting and enriching your life. The question now is, "What do you want and how are you going to get it?"

We hope we've given you some suggestions and ideas that will help you identify goals, then develop the means to reach them. Without goals, life can seem meaningless, directionless. No matter how restricted our physical health, we need long-range goals that will force us to plan for the future. How else can we attain the unattainable? That's what makes all of life's struggles worthwhile.

Remember, the enormity of your task and the degree of the reward is relative only to your resolve and ability. For some of us, just getting through the day is as much to be cheered as Franklin D. Roosevelt's presidency. The question is not, after all, "How much did you do?" Rather, it's "How well did you do?"

For the fun of it, ask yourself, "Where do I want to be ten years from now?" You'll probably be surprised at what bubbles out of your subconscious. As you sit down to plan what sort of life you want, identify your primary goal and then your secondary goal. Perhaps now, they don't seem as unattainable as they once did. We hope that, in the end, the material contained in this book contributes to your drive toward those goals, that it helps you in your everyday life, and that it adds a positive direction to your thinking.

Just remember, you really *can* can take charge of your own life, can live beyond barriers. Once you do, you'll find you've gained knowledge and understanding far beyond what you imagined possible and that you're truly the victor.

A Resource Guide for Disabled Assistance

CONTENTS

Notice

While every effort has been made to ensure the accuracy of the entries that appear in this section, neither the authors nor the publisher can make any warranty concerning any entry. Neither the authors nor the publisher assume any liability for any circumstances arising from the use of these entries.

Helplines

Here is a collection of toll-free numbers for various information centers and organizations which would be useful to have on hand.

Alzheimer's Association ....(800) 621-0379
AMC Cancer Information Center ....(800) 525-3777
American Cleft Palate Association......................(800) 242-5338
American Council of the Blind..........................(800) 424-8666
American Diabetes Association ....(800) 232-3272
American Kidney Fund....................................(800) 638-8299
American Paralysis Association ....(800) 225-0292
American Parkinson's Disease Association ....(800) 223-2732
AT&T Special Needs Center ....(800) 233-1222
           or (800) 833-3232 (TDD)
Better Hearing Institute Hearing Helpline ....(800) 424-8576
Braille Institute..(800) 252-9486
Cancer Information Service National Line ....(800) 422-6237
Civil Rights Hotline ....(800) 368-1019
Civic Information & Techniques Exchange..........(800) 223-6004
Educational Resources Information Center..........(800) 848-4815
  ERIC Clearing House on Handicapped &
  Gifted Children ....(703) 620-3660
Fair Housing and Equal Opportunity Hotline .....(800) 424-8590
Hearing Aid Helpline ....(800) 521-5247
HEATH Resource Center.................................(800) 544-3284
Hill-Burton Free Hospital Care ....(800) 638-0742
Job Accommodation Network...........................(800) 526-7234
Juvenile Diabetes Foundation International ....(800) 223-1138
           in N.Y. (800) 533-2873
Lactaid, Inc. (for lactose intolerance)................(800) 257-8650

Library of Congress National Library Service
    for Blind and Physically Handicapped..........(800) 424-9100
Lifeline Systems..(800) 451-0525
The Living Bank...(800) 528-2971
Lung Diseases ....(800) 222-5864
Medic Alert Foundation ....(800) 344-3226
                                    or (800) 432-5378
National AIDS Hotline....................................(800) 342-2437
                         or (800) 243-7889 (TTY/TDD)
National Center for the Blind
    (Job Opportunities)....................................(800) 638-7518
National Center for Stuttering..........................(800) 221-2483
National Assn. for Hearing & Speech Action
    (Voice or TDD)..(800) 638-8255
National Committee for Citizens in Education ....(800) 638-9675
National Cystic Fibrosis Foundation..................(800) 344-4823
National Down's Syndrome Society...................(800) 221-4602
National Easter Seal Society............................(800) 221-6827
National Health Information Clearinghouse ....(800) 336-4797
National Organization on Disability...................(800) 248-2253
National Organization of Social Security Claimants'
    Representatives ....(800) 431-2804
National Parkinson's Foundation.......................(800) 327-4545
National Rehabilitation Information Center ....(800) 346-2742
Organ Donor Hotline......................................(800) 243-6667
Orton Dyslexia Society ....(800) 222-3123
Practitioner's Reporting System (to report drug,
    medical device, or lab product problems) .....(800) 638-6725
RP (Retinitis Pigmentosa) Foundation Fighting
    Blindness..(800) 638-2300
Sexually Transmitted Diseases ....(800) 227-8922
Spina Bifida Association of America ....(800) 621-3141
Veterans Administration ....Call toll-free directory assistance
                (800) 555-1212 for the nearest regional office.
Vietnam Veterans of America ....(800) 424-7275
Women's Sports Foundation..............................(800) 227-3988

Organizations

For those organizations that do not list telephone numbers, information can be obtained only by writing to them. If you can't find the organization you're looking for listed here, check the listing in one of the more specialized sections.

General

AARP Fulfillment
American Association of Retired Persons
P.O. Box 2240
Long Beach, Calif. 90801

Academy of Aphasia
One Waterhouse St.
Pediatric Urology Unit
Massachusetts General Hospital
Boston, Mass. 02114
(617) 726-3877

Accessibility Information Center
National Center for a Barrier Free Environment
1140 Connecticut Ave., N.W., Suite 1006
Washington, D.C. 20036

Aid to Adopt Special Kids
450 Sansome St., Suite 210
San Francisco, Calif. 94111
(415) 434-2275

American Association for Counseling and Development
5999 Stevenson Ave.
Alexandria, Va. 22304
(703) 823-9800

American Coalition of Citizens with Disabilities
1200 15th St., N.W., Suite 201
Washington, D.C. 20005
(202) 785-4265

The American Association of Disability Communicators
2100 Pennsylvania Ave., N.W.
Washington, D.C. 20037

American Cleft Palate Association
University of Pittsburgh
1218 Grandview Ave.
Pittsburgh, Pa. 15211
(800) 242-5338
  [Provides referral index]

American Diabetes Association
1660 Duke St., National Service Center
Alexandria, Va. 22314
(800) 232-3472

American Heart Association
7320 Greenville Ave.
Dallas, Texas 75231
(214) 373-6300
  [Local chapters throughout country]

American Lung Association
1740 Broadway
New York, N.Y. 10019
(212) 315-8700
  [Local chapters throughout country]

American Orthotic and Prosthetic Association
717 Pendelton St.
Alexandria, Va. 22314
(703) 836-7116

American Paralysis Association
P.O. Box 187
Short Hills, N.J. 07078
(800) 225-0292

American Parkinson's Disease Association
60 Bay St., Suite 401
Staten Island, N.Y. 10301
(800) 223-2732

American Speech-Language-Hearing Association
10801 Rockville Pike
Rockville, Md. 20852
(800) 638-8255
  [Professional association]

Amyotrophic Lateral Sclerosis
15300 Ventura Blvd., Suite 315
Sherman Oaks, Calif. 91403
(213) 990-2150

Arthritis Foundation
1314 Spring St., N.W.
Atlanta, Ga. 30309
(404) 872-7100

Artists with Handicaps:
  Resources for Artists with Disabilities, Inc.
60 East 8th St., #289
New York, N.Y. 10003
(212) 460-8510

Association for Handicapped Students
P.O. Box 21192
Columbus, Ohio 43221
(614) 488-4972
  [Deals with postsecondary disabled]

Association for the Severely Handicapped
1600 West Armory Way
Seattle, Wash. 98119
(206) 523-8446

Asthma & Allergy Foundation
1717 Massachusetts Ave., N.W.
Washington, D.C. 20006
(202) 265-0265

Canadian Rehabilitation Council for the Disabled
Suite 2110, One Yonge St.
Toronto, Ontario
Canada M5E 1E5

Canine Companions for Independence (CCI)
P.O. Box 446
Santa Rosa, Calif. 95402-0446
(707) 528-0830
   [Nonprofit organization trains dogs to assist people with disa-
   bilities other than blindness]

Paul Levinson, President
Connected Education
92 Van Cortlandt Park South, #61
Bronx, N.Y. 10463
(212) 549-6509

Consumer Information Center
Pueblo, Colo. 81009

Cystic Fibrosis Foundation
6931 Arlington Rd.
Bethesda, Md. 20814
(800) 344-4823
   [Local chapters throughout country]

Disability Focus, Inc.
Mary Jane Owen, M.S.W., Director
1010 Vermont Ave., N.W., Suite 100
Washington, D.C. 20005
(202) 483-8582

Disabled American Veterans
P.O. Box 14301
Cincinnati, Ohio 45250
(606) 441-7300
   [Disabled American veteran employment and legislative programs]

Disabled Hotline
(800) 332-2399 8 A.M. to 4 P.M. Eastern time
   [Services such as Social Security information, college information]

Eastern Paralyzed Veterans Association
432 Park Ave. South
New York, N.Y. 10016
(212) 686-6770

ECRI
5200 Butler Pike
Plymouth Meeting, Pa. 19462
(215) 825-6000
[Tests, rates, and compares competing brands of medical devices
for health professionals. The company's highly technical reports
cost $35 to $50.]

Electronic University Network
385 8th St.
San Francisco, Calif. 94103
(800) 225-3276

Federation for Children with Special Needs
312 Stuart St.
Boston, Mass. 02116
(617) 482-2915

Friedrich's Ataxia Group in America, Inc.
P.O. Box 11116
Oakland, Calif. 94611

Goodwill Industries of America
9200 Wisconsin Ave.
Bethesda, Md. 20814
(301) 530-6500

Handicapped Organized Women, Inc.
P.O. Box 35481
Charlotte, N.C. 28235

HEATH Resource Center
   [Higher Education and the Handicapped]
Project of American Council on Education
One Dupont Circle, N.W., Suite 780
Washington, D.C. 20036
(202) 939-9320 (Voice/TDD)

Help for Incontinent People
P.O. Box 544
Union, S.C. 29379

IBM National Support Center for Persons with Disabilities
2500 Windy Ridge Parkway
Marietta, Ga. 30067
(800) 426-2133

Independent Living Research Utilization
3233 Weslayan, Suite 100
Houston, Tex. 77027
(713) 797-0200

Information Center for Individuals with Disabilities
Fort Point Place
First Floor
27-43 Wormwood St.
Boston, Mass. 02210
617-727-5540 (Voice)
1-800-462-5015 (Mass. and TTY)

Institute for International Education
890 United Nations Plaza
New York, N.Y. 10017

International Association of Laryngectomees
c/o American Cancer Society
777 Third Ave.
New York, N.Y. 10017
(212) 371-2900

International Center for the Disabled
340 East 24th St.
New York, N.Y. 10010
   [Helpful guide for those involved with employment training
   for the physically handicapped]

International Polio Network
4502 Maryland Ave.
St. Louis, Mo. 63108
(314) 361-0474

International Society for Augmentative and Alternative
  Communication
c/o Artificial Language Laboratory
Computer Science Department
Michigan State University
East Lansing, Mich. 48824

Job Accommodation Network
P.O. Box 6123
West Virginia University
Morgantown, W. Va. 26506
(800) 526-7234
  [Advises employers on adapting work areas for the disabled]

Juvenile Diabetes Foundation
432 Park Ave. South
New York, N.Y. 10016
(800) 223-1138
  [Local chapters in many states]

Leukemia Society of America
730 Third Ave.
New York, N.Y. 10017
(212) 573-8484

Lifecare
655 Aspen Ridge Dr.
Lafayette, Colo. 80026
(303) 666-9234

Mainstream Inc. and On-Call
1200 15th St., N.W.
Washington, D.C. 20036
(202) 833-1136

March of Dimes
Birth Defects Foundation
1275 Mamaroneck Ave.
White Plains, N.Y. 10605
(914) 428-7100

Meals on Wheels
[Chapters in most cities; check white pages]

Medic Alert Foundation International
Turlock, Calif. 95381-1009
(800) 432-5378

Muscular Dystrophy Association
810 Seventh Ave.
New York, N.Y. 10019
(212) 686-6770 or (212) 586-0808
[Local chapters throughout United States]

National Amputee Foundation
12-45 150th St.
Whitestone, N.Y. 11357
(718) 767-8400

National Arts and the Handicapped, Information Service
National Endowment for the Arts
1100 Pennsylvania Ave., N.W.
Washington, D.C. 20004
(202) 682-5400

National Association for Students with Handicaps
Iowa Memorial Union
University of Iowa
Iowa City, Iowa 52240

National Association of the Physically Handicapped
76 Elm St.
London, Ohio 43140
(614) 852-1664

National Ataxia Foundation
600 Twelve Oaks Center
15500 Wayzata Blvd.
Wayzata, Minn. 55391
(612) 473-7666

N.C.I. Caption Club
National Captioning Institute
c/o Public Relations Dept.
5203 Leesburg Pike
Falls Church, Va. 22041
   [Supports growth of closed captioning on television]

National Center for Youth with Disabilities
P.O. Box 721
University of Minnesota
Minneapolis, Minn. 55455
(800) 333-6293
   [Computer-accessible database for youth-related information
   about chronic or disabling conditions. Toll-free number for
   direct access, prorated hourly rate. Searches are also available
   through a voice-accessed number and the assistance of an
   information specialist.]

National Congress of Organizations of the Physically Handicapped
7611 Oakland Ave.
Minneapolis, Minn. 55423
(612) 861-2162

National Council on Independent Living (NCIL)
310 S. Peoria, Suite 201
Chicago, Ill. 60607
(312) 226-5900; (312) 226-1687 (TTY/TDD)

National Council of Independent Living Programs
c/o Max Starkloff, President
4397 Laclede Ave.
St. Louis, Mo. 63108
(314) 531-3050

National Diabetes Information Clearinghouse
Box NDIC
Bethesda, Md. 20892
(301) 468-2162

National Easter Seal Society for Crippled Children and Adults
70 East Lake St.
Chicago, Ill. 60601
(312) 726-6200
   [Local chapters in most communities]

National Health Information Clearinghouse
P.O. Box 1133
Washington, D.C. 20013-1133
(800) 336-4797

The National Home Business Network for the Disabled
P.O. Box 368
Weatherford, Tex. 76086

National Home Study Council
1601 18th St., N.W.
Washington, D.C. 20009
(202) 234-5100

National Information Center for Handicapped Children and Youth
(NICHCY)
P.O. Box 1492
Washington, D.C. 20013
(703) 893-6061

National Multiple Sclerosis Society
205 E. 42nd St.
New York, N.Y. 10017
(212) 986-3240

National Organization on Disability
910 16th St., N.W.
Washington, D.C. 20037
(202) 293-5960 or (202) 293-5968 (TDD)

National Parkinson's Foundation
1501 NW 9th Ave.
Miami, Fla. 33136
(800) 327-4545

National Rehabilitation Association
633 South Washington St.
Alexandria, Va. 22314
(703) 836-0850 (Voice/TDD)

National Rehabilitation Information Center
8455 Colesville Rd.
Silver Spring, Md. 20910
(301) 588-9284 (Voice/TDD)

National Spinal Cord Injury Association
149 California St.
Newton, Mass. 02158
(617) 964-0521

National Stroke Association
300 Hampden Ave.
Suite 240
Englewood, Colo. 80110
(303) 839-1992

National Stuttering Project
1629 7th Ave.
San Francisco, Calif. 94122
(415) 566-5324
 [Local chapters in many states]

Nebraska Polio Survivors Association
P.O. Box 37139
Omaha, Neb. 68137
 [Social Security benefits publication]

The One Shoe Crew
Georgia Hehr, R.N.
86 Clavela Ave.
Sacramento, Calif. 95828
 [National amputee group; each state has at least one amputee
 support group]

Paralyzed Veterans of America
801 18th St., N.W.
Washington, D.C. 20006
(202) 872-1300
  [Funds research, publishes legislation information; local chapters]

Parkinson's Disease Foundation
640-650 West 168th St.
New York, N.Y. 10032
(212) 923-4700

P-Polio National, Inc.
Susan Maslar
3581 University Drive
Fairfax, Va. 22030
(703) 273-8171
  [Postpolio education, support]

President's Committee on Employment of People with Disabilities
1111 20th St., N.W., Room 636
Washington, D.C. 20036
(202) 653-5044 or (202) 653-5050 (TDD)
  [On-line computerized databank]

Regional Rehabilitation Research Institute on Attitudinal, Legal,
  and Leisure Barriers
George Washington University
Barrier Awareness Project
1828 L St., N.W.
Washington, D.C. 20036

Rehabilitation Research Institute Academic Center
George Washington University
Washington, D.C. 20017
(202) 635-5822
  [Publications include booklets dealing with attitudinal barriers,
  annotated bibliographies, employment rights, recreation, and
  sexuality disability]

Sensory Technology Information Service
University of Massachusetts Medical Center
Worcester, Mass. 01605

Spina Bifida Association of America
131 Hewlett Neck Road
Woodmere, N.Y. 11598

Spinal Cord Society
Wendell Rd.
Fergus Falls, Minn. 56537
(218) 739-5252
   [Devoted to finding cure for spinal cord injury and related problems]

United Cerebral Palsy Association
2324 Forest Ave.
Staten Island, N.Y. 10303
(212) 481-6300

United Ostomy Association
1111 Wilshire Boulevard
Los Angeles, Calif. 90017

Superintendent of Documents
U.S. Government Printing Office
Washington, D.C. 20402
(202) 783-3238

Gary L. Viall
U.S. Small Business Administration
1441 L St., N.W., Room 418
Washington, D.C. 20416
(202) 653-6365 (Voice/TDD)
   [Information about loan program for disabled]

Small Business Administration Answer Desk
(800) 368-5855
   [Advice to business owners and potential owners]

Small Business Advisory Service Hotline
(800) 424-5201

Organizations for the Visually Impaired

The resources listed here for the visually impaired are not comprehensive, nor are they intended to be. Only a few are listed because the primary concentration of this book has been physical disability, and because many excellent books containing a wealth of resources for the visually impaired exist.

American Council of the Blind
1010 Vermont Ave., N.W.
Washington, D.C. 20036
(202) 393-3666

American Foundation for the Blind
15 West 16th St.
New York, N.Y. 10011
(212) 620-2000

American Printing House for the Blind
P.O. Box 6085
Louisville, Ky. 40206-0085
(502) 895-2405

Association for Education & Rehabilitation of the Blind
206 N. Washington St.
Alexandria, Va. 22314
(703) 548-1884
   [International—dedicated to advancement of education/rehabilitation of blind and visually impaired]

Blinded Veterans Association
477 H St., N.W.
Washington, D.C. 20036
(202) 371-8880
   [Helps blinded veterans with rehabilitation, vocational benefits, job placement, and other aid]

Braille Institute of America
741 North Vermont Ave.
Los Angeles, Calif. 90029
(800) 252-9486

Helen Keller National Center for Deaf-Blind Youths and Adults
111 Middle Neck Road
Sands Point, N.Y. 11050
(516) 944-8900
    [Evaluation and training for deaf-blind]

Library of Congress
National Library Service for the Blind and Physically Handi-
    capped
1291 Taylor St., N.W.
Washington, D.C. 20542
(800) 424-9100 or (202) 707-5100

National Association for Visually Handicapped
22 W. 21st St.
New York, N.Y. 10010
(212) 889-3141

National Braille Press
88 Stephen St.
Boston, Mass. 02115
(617) 266-6160
    [Computer books in braille or on cassette; newsletter]

National Federation of the Blind
1800 Johnson St.
Baltimore, Md. 21230
(301) 659-9314

Organizations for the Learning Disabled

Association for Children and Adults with Learning Disabilities
    (ACALD)
4156 Library Road
Pittsburgh, Pa. 15234
(412) 341-1515

Association for Retarded Citizens
P.O. Box 6109
Arlington, Tex. 76005
(817) 640-0204

Association of Learning Disabled Adults
P.O. Box 9722
Friendship Station
Washington, D.C. 20016

Down's Syndrome Society
145 E. 57th St.
New York, N.Y. 10022

National Network of Learning Disabled Adults
808 N. 82nd St.
Suite F2
Scottsdale, Ariz. 85257

Orton Dyslexia Society
724 York Road
Towson, Md. 21204
(800) 222-3123

Organizations for the Hearing Impaired

The resources listed here for the hearing impaired are not intended to be comprehensive; the concentration of this book has been physical disability, and many excellent books containing a wealth of resources for the hearing impaired exist.

Alexander Graham Bell Association for the Deaf, Inc.
3417 Volta Place, N.W.
Washington, D.C. 20007
(202) 337-5220 (Voice or TTY/TDD)

American Deafness and Rehabilitation Association
P.O. Box 55369
Little Rock, Ark. 72225
(501) 663-4617
   [Association of professionals who work with the deaf]

American Hearing, Language and Speech Association
10801 Rockville Pike
Rockville, Md. 20852
(301) 897-5700 (Voice or TTY/TDD)

Internal Revenue Service
(800) 428-4732 (TDD)

National Association of the Deaf
814 Thayer Ave.
Silver Spring, Md. 20910
(301) 587-1788 (Voice or TTY/TDD)

The National Information Center on Deafness
Gallaudet College
800 Florida Ave., N.E.
Washington, D.C. 20002
(202) 651-5109
   [Information about deafness, hearing loss, and Gallaudet College]

Resources for Employment and Transitional Services for the Disabled

Project Bridge
Southwest Business
Industry and Rehabilitation Assoc.
4410 N. Saddlebag Trail
Scottsdale, Ariz. 85251
(602) 949-0135

Project INTERFACE
Special Education Dept.
Arizona State Univ.
Tempe, Ariz. 85287
(602) 965-9011

Disabled Programmers, Inc.
1 West Campbell Ave.
Campbell, Calif. 95008
(408) 866-5818

Comprehensive Transition Training for Severely Handicapped
   Students
University of Colorado
School of Education
P.O. Box 7150
Colorado Springs, Colo. 80933
(303) 593-3000

School to Work Transitional Services
Conn. State Dept. of Education
P.O. Box 2219
Hartford, Conn. 06145
(203) 566-5497

Adult Basic Education Program
Gallaudet College
800 Florida Ave., N.E.
Washington, D.C. 20002
(202) 651-5000

National Transition Program Support System
National Assn. of State Directors of Special Education
1201 16th St., N.W.
Washington, D.C. 20006
(202) 822-7933

Paralyzed Veterans of America
801 18th St., N.W.
Washington, D.C. 20006
(202) 872-1300

National Rehabilitation Information Center
8455 Colesville Rd.
Silver Spring, Md. 20910
(301) 588-9284 (Voice/TDD)

International Assn. of Machinists and Aerospace Workers
National Demonstration Model for Transitional Service for
   Handicapped Youth
IAMA Apprenticeship Employment and Training Dept.
1300 Connecticut Ave., N.W.
Washington, D.C. 20036
(202) 857-5200

DVR-DPI Transitional Project
Delaware Dept. of Labor
Division of Vocational Rehabilitation
Elwyn 4th Floor
321 E. 11th St.
Wilmington, Del. 19801
(302) 571-2850

Association for Rehabilitation Programs in Data Processing
Georgia Computer Program Project
Goodwill Industries
2201 Glenwood Ave.
Atlanta, Ga. 30316
(404) 894-3972

Hawaii Transition Project
University of Hawaii
Dept. of Special Education
1776 University Ave., Wist 908
Honolulu, Hawaii 96822
(808) 948-7956

Secondary Transition and Employment Project
University of Idaho
Special Education Dept.
Moscow, Idaho 83843
(208) 885-6111

The Illinois Competitive Employment Project
University of Illinois
The Office of Career Development for Special Populations
345 Education Bldg.
1310 S. 6th St.
Champaign, Ill. 61820
(217) 333-2325

Congress of Organizations of the Physically Handicapped
16630 Beverly Ave.
Tinley Park, Ill. 60477
(312) 532-3566

Crossroads Rehabilitation Center
3242 Sutherland Ave.
Indianapolis, Ind. 46205
(317) 924-3251

Development of a Model Program to Facilitate the Transition of
  Mildly Handicapped Adolescents from Secondary to Post-
  secondary Education
University of Kansas
Learning Disabilities Research Institute
206 Carruth-O'Leary
Lawrence, Kan. 66045
(913) 864-2700

Project TRYAD: Transition Model for Multiply-Severely Handi-
  capped Young Adults
Boston College Campus School
Roberts 113
Chestnut Hill, Mass. 02167
(617) 552-8000

Maryland Rehabilitation Center
2301 Argonne Dr.
Baltimore, Md. 21218
(301) 366-8800

Community Service for Autistic Adults and Children, Inc.
751 Twinbrook Parkway
Rockville, Md. 20851
(310) 762-1650

Improving the Postsecondary Education and Employability of
  Learning Disabled Students
University of Southern Maine
Center for Research and Advanced Studies
Human Services Development Institute
246 Deering Ave.
Portland, Me. 04102
(207) 780-4141

VEConn.OR: A Model to Provide Secondary Vocational Preparation of 18–21-Year-Old Special Needs Youth
Hennepin Technical Centers
1820 N. Xenium Lane
Minneapolis, Minn. 55441
(612) 559-3535

North Dakota Dept. of Education
Capitol Bldg.
Bismark, N.D. 58505
(701) 224-2260

Transitional Employment Enterprises
1361 Elm St.
Manchester, N.H. 03101
(603) 624-0600

Las Cumbres Learning Services, Inc.
P.O. Box 663
Los Alamos, N.M. 87544
(505) 662-4323

Human Resources Center
Vocational Rehabilitation Services
I.U. Willetts Rd.
Albertson, N.Y. 11507
(516) 747-5400

Community Based Job Training for Autistic Youth
C.W. Post Campus
Long Island University
Dept. of Special Education
Greenvale, N.Y. 11548
(516) 299-0200

Undergraduate Training Program to Enhance Employment
Opportunities for Learning Disabled Students
St. Thomas Aquinas College
Route 340
Sparkill, N.Y. 10976
(914) 359-9500

Postsecondary Nonsheltered Vocational Training and Continuing
Education for Severely Handicapped Young Adults
Syracuse University
Division of Special Education and Rehabilitation
805 S. Crouse Ave.
Syracuse, N.Y. 13210
(315) 423-1870

Distributed Supported Work: A Competitive Employment Model
for Postsecondary Individuals with Severe Handicaps
University of Oregon
Specialized Training Program
Education Bldg.
Eugene, Ore. 97403
(503) 686-5311

Employability Support Network
Oregon Health Sciences University
P.O. Box 574
Portland, Ore. 97207
(503) 225-8311

Project Impact
Dallas Independent School District
Special Education Dept.
3700 Ross Ave.
Dallas, Tex. 75204
(214) 522-8220

Utah Community Based Transition
University of Utah
229 Milton Bennion Hall
Salt Lake City, Utah 84112
(801) 581-8121

American Orthotic and Prosthetic Association
717 Pendelton St.
Alexandria, Va. 22314
(703) 836-7116

Woodrow Wilson Rehabilitation Center
Fishersville, Va. 22939
(703) 885-9600

Transitional Services for Rural Students with Disabilities
American Council on Rural Special Education
Western Washington University
Bellingham, Wash. 98225
(206) 676-3000

Retail Plan for Handicapped Students on Military Installations
Clover Park School District No. 400
Resource Development and Management
10020 Gravelly Lake Dr. S.W.
Tacoma, Wash. 98499
(206) 584-9411

Association for Persons with Severe Handicaps
7010 Roosevelt Road N.E.
Seattle, Wash. 98115
(206) 523-8446

Demonstration of School Based Vocational Preparation
University of Wisconsin — Stout
Research and Training Center
Menomonie, Wis. 54751
(715) 232-1389

Specialized Equipment for Living for the Disabled

Accent Buyer's Guide
Accent Special Publications
P.O. Box 700
Bloomington, Ill. 61702
   [Good source of lists of providers of specialized equipment and
   services. Also publish a variety of publications dealing with
   practical issues concerning many different kinds of disabilities.]

Aesir Software Engineering
P.O. Box 3583
Pinedale, Calif. 93650
   [Single-switch computer software]

Alternate Stoneware
P.O. Box 2071
Charleston, W. Va. 25327-2071
(304) 346-4440
   [Stoneware made with rims that enable easier eating.]

American Stair-Glide Corporation
4001 East 138th Street
P.O. Box B
Grandview, Mo. 64080

The Anroka Collection
Box 17160
St. Paul, Minn. 55117
   [Hippacker, a large carrying bag/backpack with Velcro closures.]

AT&T National Special Needs Center
2001 Route 46
Parsippany, N.J. 07054
(800) 233-1222

Braun Corporation
1014 S. Monticello
P.O. Box 310
Winamac, Ind. 46996
(219) 946-6157
   [Swing-A-Way and Fold-A-Way Wheelchair Lifts]

Cheney Company
P.O. Box 188
2445 South Calhoun Rd.
New Berlin, Wis. 53151
   [Elevators and lifts]

Columbia Medical Manufacturing Corp.
Dept. EB
P.O. Box 633
Pacific Palisades, Calif. 90272
   [Wraparound bath support]

Consumer Care Products, Inc.
Sheboygan Falls, Wis. 53085
   [Ergonomically designed equipment. Catalog]

Custom Aid Corporation
P.O. Box 3313
Abilene, Tex. 79604
   [Custom-Aid Creeper is a lightweight frame that supports a
   child as he crawls.]

Enrichments
145 Tower Drive
P.O. Box 579
Hinsdale, Ill. 60521

Equipment Shop
P.O. Box 33
Bedford, Mass. 01730
  [Free catalog]

Everest & Jennings
3233 Mission Oaks Blvd.
Camarillo, Calif. 93010
(805) 987-6911
  [Wheelchairs]

Fashionable
99 West Street
Medfield, Mass. 02052

The Flinchbaugh Co.
390 Eberts Lane
York, Pa. 17403
  [Elevators and lifts]

Florlift of New Jersey
41 Lawrence St.
East Orange, N.J. 07017
  [Elevators and lifts]

General Electric Consumer Relations
Appliance Park
Louisville, Ky. 40225
  [Will provide a service technician to install braille controls on
  GE stoves, microwave ovens, and laundry equipment.]

GTE California, Inc.
Special Needs Center
12380 E. Firestone Blvd.
Norwalk, Calif. 90650
(800) 352-7437

Hoyle Products, Inc.
P.O. Box 606
Fillmore, Calif. 93015
  [Posture-Rite Lap Desk for bed and wheelchair]

Hydra-Fitness
P.O. Box 599
Belton, Tex. 76513-0599
(800) 433-3111
  [Fitness machines for the physically disabled]

Imex Medical, Inc.
5672 Almaden Expressway
San Jose, Calif. 95118
  [Riser Wheelchair adjusts to any position between sitting and standing]

Inclinator Company of America
Dept. 36
P.O. Box 1557
Harrisburg, Pa. 17105-1557
  [Home elevators]

International Healthcare Products, Inc.
1200 15th Street, N.W., Suite 305
Washington, D.C. 20005
(202) 659-4408
  [Bath-O-Matic]

I-Tec
5482 Business Drive, Suite C
Huntington Beach, Calif. 92649
  [Lifts]

J.L. Pachner, Ltd.
P.O. Box 164
Trabuco Cyn., Calif. 92678
  [Products to assist the disabled sportsman]

Kemp & George
2515 East 43rd St.
Chattanooga, Tenn. 37422
(800) 343-4012
  [Catalog—products for the home]

Kuschall of America
753 Calle Plano
Camarillo, Calif. 93010
  [Wheelchairs]

Maddak, Inc.
Pequannock, N.J. 07440

Mason Corporation
2605 Fessey Park Road
Nashville, Tenn. 37204
  [Therapeutic riding vehicles]

Medical Line Warehouse
P.O. Box 20609
Sarasota, Fla. 34238

Mobility Plus
215 N. 12th St.
P.O. Box 391
Santa Paula, Calif. 93060
  [Pelvic positioner]

Motions Designs, Inc.
2842 Business Park Ave.
Fresno, Calif. 93727
(209) 292-2171

New Era Transportation, Inc.
810 Moel Drive
Akron, Ohio
(800) 325-9649
  [Vans, driving adaptations, lifts, extended tops and doors, parts,
  service and repairs on all models]

Victor Passy, M.D.
4521 Campus Dr., Suite 273
Irvine, Calif. 92715
   [Valve that allows persons with tracheostomies to talk]

Prentke Romich Company
1022 Heyl Road
Wooster, Ohio 44691
(800) 262-1984
   [Communicative, environmental, and computer equipment for
   the physically handicapped]

Recreational Mobility, Inc.
P.O. Box 147
Elmira, Ore. 97347
(503) 935-2828
   [Handbike]

Royal Bee Corporation
703 Kihekah
Pawhuska, Okla. 64056
(918) 287-1044
   [Electronic Retrieve Fishing Reel designed for freshwater fishing]

Safe-T-Bath
185 Millbury Ave.
Millbury, Mass. 01527
(508) 865-2361
   [Side-opening bathtub]

Solutions
P.O. Box 6878
Portland, Ore. 97228-6878

Special Toys 4 Special Kids
11834 Wyandot Circle
Westminster, Colo. 80234
   [Toys to educate and aid development. Catalog]

STC Custom Systems
147 Eady Court
Elyria, Ohio 44035
[Transportable positioning chairs]

Street Electronics Corporation
1140 Mark Ave.
Carpinteria, Calif. 93013
(805) 684-4593
[Speech synthesizers for computers]

Swedish Rehab Catalog
100 Spence St.
Bay Shore, N.Y. 11706
(800) 645-5272
[Utensils and objects for people with limited hand use]

Technology for Independent Living, Inc.
1010 Eighth St., Suite 302
Golden, Colo. 80401
(303) 279-5447
[Apprentice II, a tabletop robotic manipulator easily interfaced
with most computers and controllable by voice command,
keyboard, or various single switches]

Ted Hoyer and Company, Inc.
P.O. Box 2744
2222 Minnesota Street
Oshkosh, Wis. 54903
[Lifts]

TherAdapt Products Inc.
17W163 Oak Lane
Bensenville, Ill. 60106
(708) 834-2461
[Pediatric equipment. Catalog]

Therapeutic Toys, Inc.
91 New Berry Road
East Haddam, Conn. 06423

Touch Turner
443 View Ridge Drive
Everett, Wash. 98203
(206) 252-1541
  [Page-turning devices]

Tumble Forms
60 Page Road
Clifton, N.J. 07012
  [Positioning seat]

Weatherproof Wheelchair Lift
P.O. Box 1308
Patterson, La. 70392

W.R. Davis Engineering Ltd.
1260 Old Innes Road
Ottawa, Ontario, Canada K1B 3V3
(613) 748-5500
  [Quick-release hand controls for automobiles]

Zygo Industries, Inc.
P.O. Box 1008
Portland, Ore. 97207-1008
(503) 684-6006

Publications

Listed below are several books and magazines dealing with various kinds of disability. The list of books, especially, is by no means exhaustive; such a task is beyond the scope of this book. For additional books dealing with disabilities, ask your local book dealer or librarian to check for you in *Books in Print*.

General publications

A Problem of Plumbing and Other Stories
by James M. Bellarosa
Susan Daniel, Sales & Marketing
John Daniel and Co. Publishers
P.O. Box 21922
Santa Barbara, Calif. 93121
(805) 962-1780

Accent on Living
Accent Special Publications
P.O. Box 700
Bloomington, Ill. 61702
(309) 378-2961

Access to the World: A Travel Guide for the Handicapped
by Louise Weiss
Henry Holt & Co., New York 1983

Aids and Appliances Review
Carroll Centre for the Blind
770 Centre St.
Newton, Mass. 02158
(617) 969-6200
  [Comprehensive overview of aids for the blind. Issue 9 and 10
  (a combined issue) deals with voice-oriented computer aids.
  Issue 11 deals with braille-oriented computer aids.]

*Alternatives: A Family Guide to Legal and Financial Planning for
the Disabled*
First Publications, Inc. 1983
1109 Garnett Place
P.O. Box 1832
Evanston, Ill. 60204

BAUD
Audio-tech Laboratories/Joe Giovanelli
1158 Stewart Ave.
Bethpage, N.Y. 11714
(516) 433-0171 (business hours only)
  [Bimonthly, cassette-only newsletter discussing microcomputer
  applications]

Beyond Rage: The Emotional Impact of Chronic Physical Illness
by Joann Lemaistre, Ph.D.
Alpine Guild
P.O. Box 183
Oak Park, Ill. 60303

Breaking New Ground Resource Manual, Vol. I
Department of Agricultural Engineering
Purdue University
West Lafayette, Ind. 47907
   [Ideas and resources from disabled farmers and ranchers]

The Catalyst
Sue Sweezey, Editor
Western Center for Microcomputers in Special Education
1259 El Camino Real, Suite 275
Menlo Park, Calif. 94025
(415) 326-6997
   [Information on recent research, hardware, software, and appli-
   cations to special education.]

Closing the Gap
P.O. Box 68
Henderson, Minn. 56044
(612) 248-3294
   [Bimonthly newsletter of computer devices]

Communication Outlook
Artificial Language Laboratory, Computer Science Dept.
Michigan State University
East Lansing, Mich. 48824
(517) 353-0870
   [Quarterly publication, international in scope, for persons with
   communication disabilities caused by neurological or neuro-
   muscular conditions]

Computer Disability News
National Easter Seal Society
Attention: Jane Minton
2023 West Ogden Ave.
Chicago, Ill. 60612

Computer Shopper
P.O. Box 1419
Titusville, Fla. 32781

Dialogue Magazine
Dialogue Publications
3132 South Oak Park Ave.
Berwyn, Ill. 60402
(312) 749-1908
[Technology and general interest magazine; flexible disks, braille or large print]

Disability Rag
P.O. Box 145
Louisville, Ky. 40201

Disability Studies Quarterly
Dr. Irving Zola, Editor
Department of Sociology
Brandeis University
Waltham, Mass. 02254

Financing Adaptive Technology: A Guide to Sources and Strategies for Blind and Visually Impaired Users
Smiling Interface
P.O. Box 2792, Church Street Station
New York, N.Y. 10008
[Guidelines useful for all disabled; cost is $23]

Guide to Adaptive Devices, Software, and Services for Special Education, Vocational Education, Vocational Rehabilitation, and Employers
by Baxter Burke, National Adviser
Special Education Programs
4111 Northside Parkway
Atlanta, Ga. 30327
[Published by IBM]

Guide to Resources for Persons with Disabilities
IBM National Support Center for Persons with Disabilities
P.O. Box 2150 (WB7F)
Atlanta, Ga. 30055
(800) 426-2133 (Contintental U.S.) or (404) 988-2733 (Ga.) or (404) 988-2729 (TDD)

Handicapped Americans Reports
Capitol Publications, Inc.
1300 North 17th St.
Arlington, Va. 22209
(703) 528-1100

Home Health Aides: How to Manage the People Who Help You
Saratoga Access Publications
Box 2346
Clifton Park, N.Y. 12065

ILRU Insights
ILRU Research and Training Center on Independent Living at
  TIRR
3400 Bissonnet, Suite 101
Houston, Tex. 77005
(713) 666-6244; (713) 666-0643 TDD

Can Do Products
Independent Living Aids, Inc.
27 East Mall
Plainview, N.Y. 11803
(800) 537-2118

Incapacitated Passengers Air Travel Guide
International Air Transport Association
200 Pearl St.
Montreal, Quebec H3A 2R4
Canada

Inside MS
National Multiple Sclerosis Society
205 East 42nd St.
New York, N.Y. 10017
(212) 986-3240

Itinerary
P.O. Box 1084
Bayonne, N.J. 07002
(201) 858-3400
  [Disabled travel magazine]

Link and Go
COPH-2
2030 West Irving Park Road
Chicago, Ill. 60618
(312) 866-8195
[Quarterly newsletter, available in print and on tape]

Mainstream
2973 Beech St.
San Diego, CA 92102
(619) 234-3138

MDA Newsmagazine
Muscular Dystrophy Association, Inc.
810 Seventh Ave.
New York, N.Y. 10019
(212) 586-0808

National Organization on Disability Report
910 16th St., N.W., Suite 600
Washington, D.C. 20006
(202) 293-5960

Oryx Press
2214 North Central at Encanto
Phoenix, Ariz. 85004
(602) 254-6156
[Directory of college facilities and services for the handicapped
has information about over 2,000 colleges and universities in the
U.S. and Canada.]

People to People Committee for the Handicapped
1111 20th St., N.W., Suite 660
Washington, D.C. 20036
(202) 653-5079
[Directory of organizations interested in the handicapped]

Publications Division
The National Mental Health Association
1021 Prince St.
Alexandria, Va. 22314-2971
[Variety of leaflets for families of the disabled]

Playback
Edward L. Potter
1308 Evergreen Ave.
Goldsboro, N.C. 27530
(919) 736-0939
[Cassette newsletter, information about audio equipment and computer aids; also sells audio equipment and supplies]

Prentke Romich Company
1022 Heyl Road
Wooster, Ohio 44691
In Ohio, call collect (216) 262-1984; others (800) 642-8255

Raised Dot Computing
Attn: David Holladay
408 South Baldwin St.
Madison, Wis. 55703
(608) 257-9595
[Personal computer applications for the blind. Both braille and audio subscriptions available.]

Rehabilitation Technology Review
RESNA
4405 East-West Highway, Suite 402
Bethesda, Md. 20814
(301) 657-4142
[Newsletter of Rehabilitation Engineering Society of North America; quarterly]

The Second Beginner's Guide to Personal Computers for the Blind
National Braille Press
88 Stephen St.
Boston, Mass. 02115
[Print, braille, or cassette copies available. National Braille Press publishes *Braille Research Newsletter*, a technical paper. NBP also has printer and modem manuals in braille and a spelling reference book on VersaBraille tape.]

Rehabilitation Gazette
Gazette International Networking Institute
4502 Maryland Ave.
St. Louis, Mo. 63108
(314) 361-0475

Sensory Aids Technology Update
399 Sherman Ave., Suite 12
Palo Alto, Calif. 94306
(415) 329-0430
    [Monthly newsletter of Sensory Aids Foundation]

Smith-Kettlewell Technical File
Smith-Kettlewell Eye Research Foundation
2232 Webster St.
San Francisco, Calif. 94115
(415) 561-1677
    [Quarterly for blind electronics professionals and hobbyists]

Social Security Disability Benefits: How to Get Them! How to Keep Them!
by James Ross
Ross Publishing Co.
Route 3
Slippery Rock, Pa. 16057

Special Times
Cambridge Development Lab
214 Third Ave.
Waltham, Mass. 02154
(800) 637-0047

Spinal Network Guide
P.O. Box 4162
Boulder, Colo. 80306
(800) 338-5412 or (303) 449-5412

Sports 'n' Spokes
Paralyzed Veterans of America
5201 No. 19th Ave., Suite 111
Phoenix, Ariz. 85015

Tactual Mapping Working Group
Australia Institute of Cartographers
GPO Box 1292
Canberra 2601, Australia
  [Quarterly newsletter]

Technical Innovations Bulletin
IRTI 26699 Snell Lane
Los Altos Hills, Calif. 94022
(415) 948-8588
  [Interviews about and demonstrations of computer and other
  technology. Also sells some appliances, audio equipment, and
  supplies.]

Together
Information Center for Individuals with Disabilities
Fort Point Place, 1st Floor
27-43 Wormwood St.
Boston, Mass. 02210
(617) 727-5540

A User's Guide to Community Entry for the Severely Handicapped
by Ernest Pancsofar and Robert Blackwell
State University of New York Press 1985
P.O. Box 6525
Ithaca, N.Y. 14850
(800) 666-2211

Voices from the Shadows: Women with Disabilities Speak Out
by Gwyneth Ferguson Matthews
Women's Educational Press
Toronto, Ontario
Canada

Ways for the Disabled
Circulation Department
C-1153
Skokie, Ill. 60076
  [Magazine for families of disabled]

With the Power of Each Breath: A Disabled Women's Anthology
edited by Susan E. Browne, Debra Conners, and Nanci Stern
Cleis Press 1985
P.O. Box 8933
Pittsburgh, Pa. 15221
(412) 731-3863

With Wings: An Anthology of Literature by and about Women with Disabilities
edited by Marsha Saxton and Florence Howe
Feminist Press 1987
311 E. 94th St.
New York, N.Y. 10128
(212) 620-3182

Learning Disabilities-Oriented Publications

A Directory of Summer Camps for Children with Learning Disabilities
ACALD, Inc. 1989
4156 Library Road
Pittsburgh, Pa. 15234
(412) 341-1515
   [Also *The College Student with a Learning Disability* and
   Directory of Educational Facilities for Learning Disabled Students]

The FCLD Resource Guide
Foundation for Children with Learning Disabilities 1985
P.O. Box 2929, Grand Central Station
New York, N.Y. 10163
(212) 687-7211

National Directory of Four-Year Colleges, Two-Year Colleges and Post-High School Training Programs for Young People with Disabilities
Partners in Publishing Company 1986
P.O. Box 50347
Tulsa, Okla. 74150
(918) 584-5906

Academics and Beyond: Volume 4, The Best of ACALD
edited by William Cruickshank and Eli Tash
Syracuse University Press
1600 Jamesville Ave.
Syracuse, N.Y. 13210

Academic Therapy Publications Parent Brochures
Academic Therapy Publications
20 Commercial Blvd.
Novato, Calif. 94947-6191

*The Basic Language Kit: A Teaching-Tutoring Aid for Adolescents
and Young Adults*
by Martin S. Weiss and Helen Ginandes Weiss
Treehouse Associates 1984
P.O. Box 1992
Avon, Colo. 81620

*College and the Learning Disabled Student: A Guide to Program
Selection, Development, and Implementation*
by Charles T. Mangrum II and Stephen S. Strichart
Grune and Stratton, Inc. 1984
6277 Sea Harbor Drive
Orlando, Fla. 32887

Fact Sheets from ACALD
20 N. Main St.
South Norwalk, Conn. 06854

Guide to College Programs for Learning Disabled Students
National Association of College Admissions Counselors 1986
9933 Lawler Ave., Suite 500
Skokie, Ill. 60077

HELDS Project Series on Teaching Learning Disabled College
Students
Educational Opportunities Program
Central Washington University
Ellensburg, Wash. 98926
(509) 963-2131

Helping Children with Specific Learning Disabilities: A Practical Guide for Parents and Teachers
by Donald H. Painting
Prentice-Hall, Inc.
Englewood Cliffs, N.J. 07632

Journal of Learning Disabilities
5615 W. Cormak Road
Cicero, Ill. 60650

The Learning Disabled Child: Ways Parents Can Help
by Suzanne H. Stevens
John F. Blair Publishing 1980
1406 Plaza Drive, S.W.
Winston-Salem, N.C. 27103

The Misunderstood Child: A Guide for Parents of of Learning Disabled Children
by Larry B. Silver
McGraw-Hill Book Company, New York 1988

No Easy Answers: The Learning Disabled Child
by Sally L. Smith
Bantam Books, Inc., New York 1985

No One to Play with: The Social Side of Learning Disabilities
by Betty B. Osman
Random House, Inc., New York 1986

A Parent's Guide to Learning Disabilities
by Alice D. D'Antoni, Darrel G. Minifie, and Elsie R. Minifie
The Continental Press, Inc.
520 E. Bainbridge St.
Elizabethtown, Pa. 17022

"Parents' Guide to 'Teacherese': A Glossary of Special Education Terms"
by Nancy O. Wilson
Special Child Publications
P.O. Box 33548
Seattle, Wash. 98133

The Powerful Parent: A Child Advocacy Handbook
by David M. Gottesman
Appleton, Century, Crofts

"Rehabilitating the Learning Disabled Adult" and "Independent Living and Learning Disabilities"
President's Committee on Employment of the Handicapped
Room 600
1111 20th St., N.W.
Washington, D.C. 20036

Reversals: A Personal Account of Victory over Dyslexia
by Eileen Simpson
Washington Square Press, New York 1981

Schooling for the Learning Disabled: A Selective Guide to LD Programs in Elementary and Secondary Schools Throughout the United States
edited by Raegene B. Pernecke and Sara M. Shreiner
SMS Publishing Corp. 1983
P.O. Box 2276
Glenview, Ill. 60025

Section 504: Help for the Learning Disabled College Student
Landmark School
Pride's Crossing, Mass. 01965

Smart but Feeling Dumb
by Harold N. Levinson
Warner Books, Inc., New York 1988

The SpecialWare Directory: A Guide to Software Sources for Special Education, 2nd edition
LINC Associates, Inc. 1985
46 Arden Road
Columbus, Ohio 43214

Specific Learning Disabilities: A Resource Manual for Vocational Rehabilitation
Vocational Rehabilitation Center 1985
1325 Forbes Ave.
Pittsburgh, Pa. 15219

Susan's Story: An Autobiographical Account of My Struggle with Dyslexia
by Susan Hampshire
St. Martin's Press, New York 1982

Their World Magazine
99 Park Ave.
New York, N.Y. 10016

Your Child Can Win
by Joan Noyes and Norma Macneill
William Morrow and Company, Inc., New York 1983

Your Child's Education: A School Guide for Parents
by Mark Wolraich, Landis Fick, and Nicholas Karagan
Charles C. Thomas Publishing 1984
2600 S. First St.
Springfield, Ill. 62717

Magazines by and for the Blind about Computers and Technology

Aids and Appliances Review
The Carroll Center for the Blind
770 Centre St.
Newton, Mass. 02158
(617) 969-6200

Apple Talk
3015 S. Tyler St.
Little Rock, Ark. 72204
(501) 666-6552 (6–9 P.M. CST only)

BAUD (Blind Apple Users' Discussion)
Audio-Tech Laboratories
1158 Stewart Ave.
Bethpage, N.Y. 11714
(516) 433-0171

Playback
1308 Evergreen Ave.
Goldsboro, N.C. 27530
(919) 734-9173

Raised Dot Computing
Raised Dot Computing, Inc.
408 S. Baldwin St.
Madison, Wis. 53703

Sensus
Sensory Aids Foundation
399 Sherman Ave., Suite 12
Palo Alto, Calif. 94306
(415) 329-0430

Smith-Kettlewell Technical File
Rehabilitation Engineering Center
The Smith-Kettlewell Eye Research Foundation
2232 Webster St.
San Francisco, Calif. 94115
(415) 561-1619

Tactic
Clovernook Printing House for the Blind
7000 Hamilton Ave.
Cincinnati, Ohio 45231
(513) 522-3860

Technical Innovations Bulletin
Innovative Rehabilitation Technology, Inc.
26699 Snell Lane
Los Altos Hills, Calif. 94022
(415) 948-8588

*In addition, various foundations and organizations for the blind listed in
the Organizations section of this appendix publish general-interest newsletters and magazines by and for the blind.*

Special Needs Catalogs

AT&T Special Needs Center
2001 Route 46, Suite 310
Parsippany, N.J. 07054
(800) 233-1222

Accent Buyer's Guide
Accent Special Publications
P.O. Box 700
Bloomington, Ill. 61702

Access to Recreation
2509 E. Thousand Oaks Blvd., Suite 430
Thousand Oaks, Calif. 91360
(800) 634-4351 or (805) 498-7535
   [Catalog of adaptive recreation equipment]

Adaptive Communication Systems, Inc.
P.O. Box 12440
Pittsburgh, Pa. 15231
(412) 264-2288
   [Computer communication equipment]

Bristol-Myers Co.
Guide to Consumer Product Information
P.O. Box 14177
Baltimore, Md. 21268
   [Personal care, household, medical and pain treatment resources]

Consumer Care Products, Inc.
Sheboygan Falls, Wis. 53085
   [Ergonomically designed equipment]

Consumer's Guide to Toll-Free Hotlines
P.O. Box 19405
Washington, D.C. 20036
   [Ralph Nader booklet; cost is $1]

Dorothy O'Callaghan
P.O. Box 19083
Washington, D.C. 20036
  [Directory of more than 200 mail-order catalogs specializing in
  the particular needs of the disabled]

Equipment Shop
P.O. Box 33
Bedford, Mass. 01730

Heidico Inc.
P.O. Box 3170
Blaine, Wash. 98230

Hydra-Fitness
P.O. Box 599
Belton, Texas 76513-0599
(800) 433-3111
  [Fitness machines for the physically disabled]

IBM National Support Center for Persons with Disabilities
2500 Windy Ridge Parkway
Marietta, Ga. 30067
(800) 426-2133

Kemp & George
2515 E. 43rd St.
Chattanooga, Tenn. 37422
(800) 343-4012
  [Products for the home]

MARC Mercantile, Ltd.
Div., HAC Box 3055
Kalamazoo, Mich. 49003
(800) 445-9968 (Voice) or (616) 381-2219 (TDD)
  [Special needs catalog for hearing-impaired]

J.L. Pachner, Ltd.
33012 Lighthouse Court
San Juan Capistrano, Calif. 92675
  [Products to assist the disabled sportsman]

Radio Shack Catalog for People with Special Needs
At local Radio Shack stores or from:
300 One Tandy Center
Fort Worth, Tex. 76102

Sears Home Health Care Products Specialog
Sears, Roebuck and Co.
3333 W. Arthington St.
Chicago, Ill. 60607
   [Order by phoning nearest Sears catalog store]

Sonic Alert
209 Voorheis
Pontiac, Mich. 48053
(313) 858-8957 (Voice/TDD)
   [Products for hearing-impaired]

Special Toys 4 Special Kids
11834 Wyandot Circle
Westminster, Colo. 80234
   [Toys to educate and aid development]

Stuart's Sport Specialties
7081 Chad St.
Anchorage, Alaska 99502
(907) 349-8377
   [Outdoors catalog]

Swedish Rehab
100 Spence St.
Bay Shore, N.Y. 11706
(800) 645-5272
   [Utensils and objects for people with limited hand use]

TherAdapt Products, Inc.
17W163 Oak Lane
Bensenville, Ill. 60106
   [Pediatric equipment]

Ways and Means
The Capability Collection
28001 Citrin Drive
Romulus, Mich. 48174
(800) 654-2345
  [General catalog]

Woodworker's Catalog
The Woodworker's Store
21801 Industrial Blvd.
Rogers, Minn. 55374
(612) 428-2199

Computers, Software, and Gadgets

Adaptive Communication Systems, Inc.
P.O. Box 12440
Pittsburgh, Pa. 15231
(412) 264-2288
  [Long Range Optical Pointer (LROP), used as a head pointer
  for persons who cannot operate a standard computer keyboard]

Aesir Software Engineering
P.O. Box 3583
Pinedale, Calif. 93650
  [Single switch computer software]

Aids and Appliances Review
Carroll Centre for the Blind
770 Centre St.
Newton, Mass. 02158
(617) 969-6200
  [Comprehensive overview of aids for the blind. Issue 9 and 10
  (a combined issue) deals with voice-oriented computer aids.
  Issue 11 deals with braille-oriented computer aids.]

American West Engineering
2144 S. 1100 East, Suite 150
Salt Lake City, Utah 84106

[Multimouse, single-handed data entry device for IBM computers, ideal for persons with use of only one hand. By pressing two or more buttons on the palm-shaped chord keyboard, all the keys on a standard IBM keyboard can be emulated. Available for right or left hand.]

Apollo Electronic Visual Aids
P.O. Box 2755
2932 Lassen St.
Chatsworth, Calif. 91311
(213) 700-2666
[Large-print computer terminal and typing system]

Arts Computer Products
145 Tremont St., Suite 407
Boston, Mass. 02111
(617) 482-8248
[Large-print terminal, talking terminal]

Assistive Device Database System (ADDS)
American Information Data Search, Inc.
2326 Fair Oaks Blvd., Suite C
Sacramento, Calif.
(916) 925-4554 (modem)
[Write for information before calling]

BAUD (Blind Apple Users' Discussion)
Audio-tech Laboratories, Joe Giovanelli
1158 Stewart Ave.
Bethpage, N.Y. 11714
(516) 433-0171
[Bimonthly, cassette-only newsletter discussing microcomputer applications; emphasis on Apple software and Computer Aids, Inc. products.]

Arnold Balliet
Cascade Graphics Development
1000 South Grand Ave.
Santa Ana, Calif. 92705
(714) 474-6200

[Cash III Voice Controlled System enables people with limited or no use of their hands to operate programs by voice, including using the telephone, turning pages, turning on a light, and opening a door.]

The Catalyst
Western Center for Microcomputers in Special Education
1259 El Camino Real, Suite 275
Menlo Park, Calif. 94025
(415) 326-6997
[Information on recent research, hardware, software, and applications to special education]

Clark Technologies
Mr. Lee Brown
16205 Fantasia Drive
Tampa, Fla. 33623
(813) 962-4105 or 223-8155
[Braillink paperless brailler and a talking terminal]

Closing the Gap
5139 Wentworth Ave. S.
Minneapolis, Minn. 55419
(612) 665-6573
[Bimonthly newsletter]

ComputAbility Corp.
101 Route 46
Pine Brook, N.J. 07058
[Complete Apple or IBM computer systems for the disabled]

Computer Shopper
P.O. Box 1419
Titusville, Fla. 32781

Cyberon Corp.
Eliot Friedman
1175 Wendy Road
Ann Arbor, Mich. 48103
(313) 994-0326
[Cybertalker speech terminal, Apple Cyber Card]

Designing Aids for Disabled Adults (DADA)
1024 Dupont St.
Unit 5
Toronto, Ontario M6H 2A2
Canada
(416) 533-4494
[PC A.I.D. makes IBM computers more accessible to persons with physical disabilities. With PC A.I.D. the computer can be operated with a single switch.]

Electronic Specialties
5230 Girard Ave. North
Minneapolis, Minn. 55430
(612) 521-0008
[AVOS System: hardware is Osborne 1 or Zorba Computer with speech output; software includes word processing, database, and communications programs.]

Enable Software
Robert Artusy
2340 Martin Luther King Jr. Way, Suite B
Berkeley, Calif. 94704
(415) 540-0389
[Talking software for Radio Shack Models 3 and 4 and for the Kaypro; for screen review and for word processing]

Hadley School for the Blind
700 Elm Street
Winnetka, Ill. 60093
(800) 323-4238; in Illinois, (312) 446-8111
[Home-study computer literacy course]

Hy-Tek Manufacturing Inc.
412 Bucktail Lane
Sugar Grove, Ill. 60554
(312) 466-7664
[Voice Interactive Computer System (V.I.C.). IBM-compatible, also features voice output and is available in three basic CPU configurations.]

IBM Voice Communication Option
IBM Corp.
National Support Center for Persons with Disabilities
2500 Windy Ridge Parkway
Marietta, Ga. 30067
(800) 426-2133

Intelligent Modem
Phone-TTY, Inc.
202 Lexington Ave.
Hackensack, N.J. 07601
(201) 489-7889 (Voice or TTY)

Maryland Computer Services, Inc.
2010 Rock Spring Road
Forest Hill, Md. 21050
(301) 879-3366
   [Total Talk PC, I.T.S. (Information Through Speech) computer,
   Total Talk 2 speech terminal and the Cranmer Modified Perkins
   Brailler, a hard-copy braille terminal suitable for individual and
   classroom use. Also the Thiel braille printer and the Ready
   Reader, which scans typed materials in selected fonts and sends
   its output to a computer.]

National Braille Press
88 Stephen Street
Boston, Mass. 02115
(617) 266-6160
   [Various publications, including those dealing with computers
   and the blind.]

National Easter Seal Society
Attention: Jane Minton
70 Eastlake St.
Chicago, Ill. 60601
(312) 726-6200
   [*Computer Disability News* newsletter]

Elliot M. Schreier, Director
National Technology Center, American Foundation for the Blind
15 West 16th St.
New York, N.Y. 10011
(212) 620-2080
[Information about large print for PC]

Playback
Edward L. Potter
1308 Evergreen Ave.
Goldsboro, N.C. 27530
(919) 736-0939
[Cassette newsletter, information about audio equipment and computer aids]

Psycho-linguistic Research Associates
2055 Sterling Ave.
Menlo Park, Calif. 94025
(415) 854-1771
[Hardware and software for talking Zenith Heathkit Computer and software for speech in Radio Shack computers]

Raised Dot Computing
Attn: David Holladay
408 South Baldwin St.
Madison, Wis. 55703
(608) 257-9595
[Personal computer applications for the blind. Both braille and audio subscriptions available.]

Softwarehouse
3080 Olcott Dr., Suite 125A
Santa Clara, Calif. 95054
(408) 748-0461
[SLICworks, an IBM-compatible PC program. Shareware product, which means a user can purchase it on disk and try the program before registering. For more information and free catalog of other products contact Softwarehouse.]

Special Times
Cambridge Development Lab
214 Third Ave.
Waltham, Mass. 02154
(800) 637-0047
   [Primarily for parents/teachers of children with learning or problem-solving skills.]

Street Electronics Corporation
6420 Villa Real
Carpinteria, Calif. 93013
(805) 684-4593
   [Speech synthesizers for computers]

Technical Innovations Bulletin
IRTI 26699 Snell Lane
Los Altos Hills, Calif. 94022
(415) 948-8588
   [Interviews about and demonstrations of computer and other technology]

Trace Center
The Waisman Center
University of Wisconsin/Madison
1500 Highland Ave.
Madison, Wis. 53705
(608) 262-6966
   [Registry of software for disabled, workshops on computer access]

Vtek (formerly Visualtek)
1735 W. Rosecrans Ave.
Gardena, Calif. 90249
(213) 329-3463
   [Large-print computer access devices for Apple and IBM PC]

Specialized Computer Software

AARON
AESIR Software Engineering
P.O. Box 5383
Pinedale, Calif. 93650
 [Word processor anticipates words]

Hartley Courseware, Inc.
133 Bridge St.
Dimondale, Mich. 48821
(517) 646-6458
 [Instructional programs]

Electronic 31-Day Calendar
Computer Users of America
5028 Merit Drive
Flint, Mich. 48506
 [With voice]

IBM Augmented Phone Services
IBM Corp.
National Support Center for Persons with Disabilities
2500 Windy Ridge Parkway
Marietta, Ga. 30067
(800) 426-2133

Lambert Software Co.
P.O. Box 1257
Ramona, Calif. 92065
(619) 789-1438
 [Instructional/retraining software]

Listen to Learn
IBM Corp.
IBM Direct, PC Software Dept.
One Culver Road
Dayton, N.J. 08810
 [Word processor with voice]

Micro-Interpreter I "The Finger-speller"
Edu Tec, Inc.
  (formerly Microtech Consulting Company, Cedar Falls, Iowa)
7070 Brooklyn Blvd.
Minneapolis, Minn. 53005
(414) 784-8075

PC-Fingers
Midwest Health Programs, Inc.
408 West Vermont
P.O. Box 3023
Urbana, Ill. 61801
(217) 367-5293

Prompt-Writer
Syn-Talk Systems & Services
70 Estero Avenue
San Francisco, Calif. 94127
  [Word processor with voice]

Rapsheet
BAUD
337 S. Peterson
Louisville, Ky. 40206
  [Spreadsheet with voice]

Special Education Software Center
3857 North High Street
Columbus, Ohio 43214
(800) 327-5892

TDD Emulation
Phone-TTY, Inc.
202 Lexington Avenue
Hackensack, N.J. 07601
(201) 489-7889 (Voice or TTY/TDD)

Tele-Talk
Computer Users of America
5028 Merit Drive
Flint, Mich. 48506
  [Phone/address list with voice]

ThinkTank
Living Videotext Inc.
2432 Charleston Road
Mountain View, Calif. 94043
  [Outliner]

Word Talk
Computer Aids Corp.
4320 Stevens Creek Blvd., Suite 290
San Jose, Calif. 95129
  [Word processor with voice]

Computer Bulletin Boards for the Disabled

Computer Bulletin Board Systems (BBSs) come and go as their operators have time to run them. These are a few of the many around the country that have been on-line for an extended period of time. Nearly every one will have numbers of others you can call.

4-Sights Network ....(313) 272-7111*
Accent on Information (Equipment Information) (309) 378-2961
Atlanta PC User Group BBS ....(404) 988-2790
The Braille Board..(904) 433-5325
Bullet-80 ....(203) 629-4375
Capital Telecom64 ....(518) 436-1422
Care Net BBS ....(219) 233-1261
Computer Clinic...(919) 834-0649
COPH-2 BBS. ....(312) 286-0608
Direct Link..(805) 964-5708
Disabled Interest Group's Electronic Exchange....(619) 454-8078
Disabled Children's Computer Group BBS ....(415) 642-7387
Disabled Interest Group—El Paso.....................(915) 592-5424
Dr. Ross Shuping's BBS ....(919) 756-3369
DxNet ....(800) 648-0069
Florida Information Resources Network.............(904) 487-1078
Handicapped Information Exchange ....(408) 462-2692
Handicapped Educational Exchange..................(301) 593-7033
                                        In Texas (512) 383-5860

Host BBS ....(518) 793-9574
IBM Support Center..(800) 426-2133
Info-80 ....(215) 434-2237†
Insight ....(301) 543-2146
Kendall Net (Hearing Impaired) ....(202) 651-5260
Mailbox...(612) 638-4703
Moore (N.J.) School.......................................(201) 547-3208
National Council of Independent Living ....(918) 587-4493
New York On Line...(718) 852-2662
Office of Education Research and Improvement...(800) 222-4922
San Diego State Univ. Educational Technology ....(619) 265-3428
Sector ....(801) 750-2032
Sounding Board...(412) 363-9937
SPINE BBS (Northwestern Memorial Hospital)...(312) 908-2583
Trace Center (Univ. of Wisconsin)....................(608) 262-2966

* *Charges a fee*
†*1,200 baud only*

Airline Toll-Free Numbers

To help you plan your traveling yourself, here are the toll-free numbers for nearly every airline that takes off and lands in the United States. Domestic (U.S.-based) airlines are listed first, followed by foreign carriers. These numbers change frequently. If you have trouble reaching a number, call WATS information at (800) 555-1212.

Domestic

AAA Air Ambulance..(800) 245-9987
Aero Coach Aviation ....(800) 327-0010
Air Cal ....(800) 424-7225
Air Midwest..(800) 835-2953
Air Nevada...(800) 634-6377
Alaska Airlines ....(800) 426-0333
Allegheny Commuter.......................................(800) 428-4253
Aloha Airlines ....(800) 367-5250
Alpha Air...(800) 421-9353

Ambassadair..(800) 225-9919
America West Airlines...(800) 247-5692
American Airlines ....(800) 433-7300
          or (800) 446-7834
American Transair ....(800) 225-9920
Aspen Airways ....(800) 241-6522
Associated Airlines..(800) 227-7110
Beaver Aviation...(800) 245-3248
Braniff ....(800) 272-6433
         TDD (800) 356-3889
Britt Airways ....(800) 652-7488
Cayman Airways...(800) 422-9626
Comair Airlines..(800) 354-9822
Continental Airlines ....(800) 525-0280
Delta Airlines...(800) 221-1212
Direct Air Inc ....(800) 428-0706
Eastern Airlines ....(800) 327-8376
Gulf Air...(800) 223-1740
Hawaiian Airlines...(800) 367-5320
Horizon Air ....(800) 547-9308
Martinair ....(800) 282-3828
Mesa Air Shuttle..(800) 637-2247
Midway Airlines ....(800) 621-5700
Midwest Express...(800) 452-2022
New England Airline...(800) 243-2460
New York Air ....(800) 525-0280
Northwest Airlines..(800) 225-2525
Northwest Orient ....(800) 447-4747
Olympic Airways..(800) 223-1226
Pan American...(800) 221-1111
Reeve Aleutian ....(800) 544-2248
Rynes Aviation ....(800) 621-4110
Scenic Airlines..(800) 634-6801
Sky West Airlines..(800) 453-9417
Southwest Airlines...(800) 531-5601
Trans World Airlines..(800) 221-2000
Tower Air..(800) 221-2500
Trans Colorado..(800) 525-0280

US Air..(800) 428-4322
United Airlines..................................(800) 241-6522
Virgin Air..(800) 522-3084
WRA Air Service ....(800) 334-5890

Foreign

ALM Antilean Airline........................(800) 327-7230
Aer Lingus ....(800) 223-7660
Aero Peru..(800) 255-7378
Aeromexico ....(800) 237-6639
Air Canada..(800) 422-6232
Air France ....(800) 237-2747
Air India...(800) 223-7776
Air Jamaica.......................................(800) 523-5585
Air New Zealand...............................(800) 262-1234
Alia Royal Jordanian ....(800) 223-0470
Alitalia...(800) 223-5730
Australian Airlines ....(800) 922-5122
Aviateca..(800) 327-9832
Bahamas Air ....(800) 222-4262
British Airways.................................(800) 247-9297
Canadian Airlines International..........(800) 426-7000
Czechoslovak Air..............................(800) 223-2365
Dominicana Airlines ....(800) 327-7240
Ecuatoriana.......................................(800) 328-2367
El Al Israel.......................................(800) 223-6700
Ethiopian Airlines ....(800) 433-9677
                                        or (800) 445-2733
Faucett Peruvian ....(800) 327-3368
Guyana Airways ....(800) 327-8680
Japan Airlines ....(800) 525-3663
KLM Dutch Airlines ....(800) 777-5553
Korean Air ....(800) 421-8200
LAN Chile Airlines...........................(800) 327-3360
LAP Aer Paraguayas..........................(800) 327-3551
LOT Polish Airlines ....(800) 223-0593

Lacsa	(800) 225-2272
Lloyd Aero Boliviano	(800) 327-7407
Lufthansa	(800) 645-3880
Malev Hungarian Air	(800) 223-6884
Mexicana	(800) 531-7921
Nigeria Airways	(800) 223-1070
Pakistan International	(800) 221-2552
Philippine Airlines	(800) 435-9725
Qantas Airlines	(800) 227-4500
Royal Air Maroc	(800) 292-0081
Sabena	(800) 645-1382
SAS Scandinavian	(800) 221-2350
Saudi Arabian	(800) 472-8342
Singapore Airlines	(800) 742-3333
South African Air	(800) 722-9675
Swissair	(800) 221-6644
TAP Air Portugal	(800) 221-7370
Taca International	(800) 535-8780
Tan-Sahsa Honduras	(800) 327-1225
Thai Airways	(800) 426-5204
US Air	(800) 251-5720
Varig Brasilian	(800) 468-2744
Viasa-Venezuelian	(800) 327-5454
Yemen Airways	(800) 257-1133

Tourist Information Offices

Listed here are the addresses of the tourist information offices for most countries that have them in the United States. For a packet of information, merely write or call the appropriate office and ask for general tourist information.

Antigua
Antigua Department of Tourism & Trade
610 Fifth Ave., Suite 311
New York, N.Y. 10020
(212) 541-4117

Argentina
Argentina Tourist Information
330 West 58th St., Suite 6K
New York, N.Y. 10019
(212) 765-8833

Aruba
Aruba Tourism Authority
1270 Avenue of the Americas, Suite 2212
New York, N.Y. 10020
(212) 246-3030

Australia
Australian Tourist Commission
2121 Avenue of the Stars, Suite 1200
Los Angeles, Calif. 90067
(213) 552-1988

Austria
Austrian National Tourist Office
11601 Wilshire Blvd., Suite 2480
Los Angeles, Calif. 90025
(213) 477-3332

Bahamas
Bahamas Tourist Office
3450 Wilshire Blvd., Suite 208
Los Angeles, Calif. 90010
(213) 385-0033

Barbados
Barbados Board of Tourism
800 Second Ave., 17th Floor
New York, N.Y. 10017
(212) 986-6516

Belgium
Belgian National Tourist Office
745 Fifth Ave., Suite 714
New York, N.Y. 10151
(212) 758-8130

Bermuda
Bermuda Department of Tourism
310 Madison Ave., Suite 201
New York, N.Y. 10017
(212) 818-9800

Bonaire
Bonaire Government Tourist Office
275 Seventh Ave., 19th Floor
New York, N.Y. 10001-6788
(212) 242-7707

Brazil
Brazilian Trade Center, Tourist Information
3810 Wilshire Blvd., Suite 1500
Los Angeles, Calif. 90010
(213) 382-3133

British Columbia
Government of British Columbia Trade & Tourism
2600 Michelson Drive, Suite 1050
Irvine, Calif. 92715
(800) 663-6000 or (714) 852-1054

British Virgin Islands
British Virgin Islands Tourist Board
370 Lexington Ave., Suite 511
New York, N.Y. 10017
(800) 835-8530

Bulgaria
Balkan Holidays Tourist Information
161 East 86th St., 2nd Floor
New York, N.Y. 10028
(212) 722-1110

Canada
Canadian Consulate General, Tourist Information
300 S. Grand Ave., 10th Floor
Los Angeles, Calif. 90071
(213) 687-7432

Caribbean
Caribbean Tourism Organization
20 East 46th St., 4th Floor
New York, N.Y. 10017
(212) 682-0435

Cayman Islands
Cayman Islands Department of Tourism
3440 Wilshire Blvd., Suite 1202
Los Angeles, Calif. 90010
(213) 738-1969

Chile
Chilean National Tourist Board
510 West 6th St., Suite 1210
Los Angeles, Calif. 90014
(213) 627-4293

China
China National Tourist Office
333 W. Broadway, Suite 201
Glendale, Calif. 91204
(818) 545-7505

Colombia
Colombian Government Tourist Office
140 East 57th St., 2nd Floor
New York, N.Y. 10022
(212) 688-0151

Costa Rica
Costa Rica Tourist Board
3540 Wilshire Blvd., Suite 707
Los Angeles, Calif. 90010
(213) 382-8080

Curaçao
Curaçao Tourist Board
400 Madison Ave., Suite 311
New York, N.Y. 10017
(212) 751-8266

Cyprus
Cyprus Tourism Organization
13 East 40th St., 3rd Floor
New York, N.Y. 10016
(212) 213-9100

Czechoslovakia
Cedok, Tourist Information
10 East 40th St., Suite 1902
New York, N.Y. 10016
(212) 689-9720

Denmark
Danish Tourist Board
75 Rockefeller Plaza
New York, N.Y. 10019
(212) 582-2802

Dominican Republic
Dominican Tourist Information Center
485 Madison Ave., Suite 202
New York, N.Y. 10022
(212) 826-0750

Ecuador
Ecuadorian Consulate, Tourist Information
548 S. Spring St.
Los Angeles, Calif. 90013
(213) 628-3014

Egypt
Egyptian Tourist Authority
323 Geary St., Suite 303
San Francisco, Calif. 94102
(415) 781-7676

Fiji
Fiji Visitors Bureau
6151 W. Century Blvd.
Los Angeles, Calif. 90045
(213) 417-2234

Finland
Finnish Tourist Board
655 Third Ave.
New York, N.Y. 10017
(212) 370-5540

France
French Government Tourist Office
9454 Wilshire Blvd., Suite 303
Beverly Hills, Calif. 90212
(213) 271-2665 or (213) 272-2661

French Guiana
(*See* French Government Tourist Office)

West Germany
German National Tourist Office
444 S. Flower St., Suite 2230
Los Angeles, Calif. 90071
(213) 688-7332

Great Britain
British Tourist Authority
350 S. Figueroa St., Suite 450
Los Angeles, Calif. 90071
(213) 628-3525

Greece
Greek National Tourist Organization
611 West 6th St., Suite 1998
Los Angeles, Calif. 90017
(213) 626-6696

Grenada
Grenada Tourist Information Office
141 East 44th St., Suite 701
New York, N.Y. 10017
(212) 687-9554

Guadeloupe
(*See* French Government Tourist Office)

Guatemala
Guatemala Tourist Commission
2216 Coral Way
Miami, Fla. 33145
(305) 854-1544

Haiti
Haiti Government Tourist Bureau
488 Madison Ave., Room 1505
New York, N.Y. 10022
(212) 697-9767

Hong Kong
Hong Kong Tourist Assn.
10940 Wilshire Blvd., Suite 1220
Los Angeles, Calif. 90024
(213) 208-4582

Hungary
Hungarian Travel Bureau
1 Parker Plaza, Room 1104
Ft. Lee, N.J.
(212) 582-7412 or (201) 592-8585

Iceland
(*See* Scandinavia)

India
Government of India Tourist Office
3550 Wilshire Blvd., Suite 204
Los Angeles, Calif. 90010
(213) 380-8855

Indonesia
Indonesia Tourist Promotion Board
3457 Wilshire Blvd.
Los Angeles, Calif. 90010
(213) 387-2078

Ireland
Irish Tourist Board
757 Third Ave., 19th Floor
New York, N.Y. 10017
(212) 418-0800

Israel
Israel Government Tourist Office
6380 Wilshire Blvd., Suite 1700
Los Angeles, Calif. 90048
(213) 658-7462

Italy
Italian Government Travel Office
360 Post St., Suite 801
San Francisco, Calif. 94108
(415) 392-6206

Ivory Coast
Ivory Coast Tourist Bureau
2424 Massachusetts Ave.
Washington, D.C. 20008
(202) 797-0300

Jamaica
Jamaica Tourist Board
3440 Wilshire Blvd., Suite 1207
Los Angeles, Calif. 90010
(213) 384-1123

Japan
Japan National Tourist Organization
624 S. Grand Ave., Suite 2640
Los Angeles, Calif. 90017
(213) 623-1952

Jordan
Jordan Information Bureau
2319 Wyoming Ave., N.W.
Washington, D.C. 20008
(202) 265-1606

Kenya
Kenya Tourist Office
9100 Wilshire Blvd., Suite 111
Beverly Hills, Calif. 90212
(213) 274-6635

Korea
Korea National Tourism Corp.
510 West 6th St., Suite 323
Los Angeles, Calif. 90014
(213) 623-1226

Luxembourg
Luxembourg Tourist Office
801 Second Ave.
New York, N.Y. 10017
(212) 370-9850

Macao
Furman Communications Inc., Tourist Information
P.O. Box 1860
Los Angeles, Calif. 90078
(213) 851-3402

Malaysia
Malaysian Tourist Information Center
818 West 7th St.
Los Angeles, Calif. 90017
(213) 689-9702

Malta
Consulate of Malta, Tourist Information
249 East 35th St.
New York, N.Y. 10016
(212) 725-2345

Martinique
(*See* French Government Tourist Office)

Mauritius
Mauritius Tourist Information Service
15 Penn Plaza, 415 7th Ave.
New York, N.Y. 10001
(212) 239-8350

Mexico
Mexican Government Tourism Office
10100 Santa Monica Blvd., Suite 224
Los Angeles, Calif. 90067
(213) 203-8191

Monaco
Monaco Government Tourist Office
845 Third Ave.
New York, N.Y. 10022
(212) 759-5227

Morocco
Moroccan National Tourist Office
421 N. Rodeo Drive, Second Floor
Beverly Hills, Calif. 90210
(213) 271-8939

Netherlands
Netherlands Board of Tourism
90 New Montgomery St., Suite 305
San Francisco, Calif. 94105
(415) 543-6772

Netherlands Antilles
St. Maarten Tourist Office
275 Seventh Ave., 19th Floor
New York, N.Y. 10001
(212) 989-0000

New Zealand
New Zealand Tourist & Publicity Office
10960 Wilshire Blvd., Suite 1530
Los Angeles, Calif. 90024
(213) 477-8241

Norway
(*See* Scandinavia)

Pacific Asia
Pacific Asia Travel Assn.
1 Montgomery St.
Telesis Tower, Suite 1750
San Francisco, Calif. 94104
(415) 986-4646

Panama
Panama Consul General, Tourist Information
548 S. Spring St., Suite 1040
Los Angeles, Calif. 90013
(213) 627-9139

Papua New Guinea
Air Niugini Office, Tourist Information
5000 Birch St., Suite 3000, West Tower
Newport Beach, Calif. 92660
(714) 752-5440

Paraguay
Paraguay Embassy, Tourist Information
2400 Massachusetts Ave., N.W.
Washington, D.C. 20008
(202) 483-6962

Peru
Peru Tourist Office
999 S. Bayshore Drive, Suite 201
Miami, Fla. 33131
(305) 374-0023

Philippines
Philippine Department of Tourism
3460 Wilshire Blvd., Suite 1212
Los Angeles, Calif. 90010
(213) 487-4525

Poland
Orbis Polish Travel Bureau
500 Fifth Ave.
New York, N.Y. 10110
(212) 391-0844

Portugal
Portuguese National Tourist Office
590 Fifth Ave.
New York, N.Y. 10036
(212) 354-4403

Puerto Rico
Puerto Rico Tourism Co.
3575 W. Cahuenga Blvd., Suite 248
Los Angeles, Calif. 90068
(213) 874-5991

Quebec
Quebec Government Office, Tourist Information
700 S. Flower St., Suite 1520
Los Angeles, Calif. 90017
(213) 689-4861

Romania
Romanian National Tourist Office
573 Third Ave.
New York, N.Y. 10016
(212) 697-6971

Russia (USSR)
Intourist Travel Information Office in the USA
630 Fifth Ave., Suite 868
New York, N.Y. 10111
(212) 757-3884

St. Lucia
St. Lucia Tourist Board
820 Second Ave., 9th Floor
New York, N.Y. 10017
(212) 867-2950

St. Vincent, Grenadines
St. Vincent, Grenadines Tourist Office
801 Second Ave., 21st Floor
New York, N.Y. 10017
(212) 687-4981

Samoa
Western Samoa Trade & Tourism Office
465 Kapahulu Ave., Suite 2-H
Honolulu, Hawaii 96815
(808) 734-2711

Scandinavia
Scandinavian National Tourist Offices
655 Third Ave., 18th Floor
New York, N.Y. 10017
(212) 949-2333

Seychelles
Seychelles Tourist Office
P.O. Box 33018
St. Petersburg, Fla. 33733
(813) 864-3013

Singapore
Singapore Tourist Promotion Board
8484 Wilshire Blvd., Suite 510
Beverly Hills, Calif. 90211
(213) 852-1901

South Africa
South African Tourism Board
Suite 1524, 9841 Airport Blvd.
Los Angeles, Calif. 90045
(213) 641-8444

Spain
National Tourist Office of Spain
8383 Wilshire Blvd., Suite 960
Beverly Hills, Calif. 90211
(213) 658-7188

Sri Lanka
Sri Lanka Tourist Board
2148 Wyoming Ave., N.W.
Washington, D.C. 20008
(202) 483-4025

Sweden
(*See* Scandinavia)

Switzerland
Swiss National Tourist Office
250 Stockton St.
San Francisco, Calif. 94108
(415) 362-2260

Tahiti
Tahiti Tourist Board
12233 W. Olympic Blvd., Suite 110
Los Angeles, Calif. 90064
(213) 207-1919

Taiwan
Republic of China Tourism Bureau
166 Geary St., Suite 1605
San Francisco, Calif. 94108
(415) 989-8677

Tanzania
Tanzania Mission
205 East 42nd St., Room 1300
New York, N.Y. 10017
(212) 972-9160

Thailand
Tourism Authority of Thailand
3440 Wilshire Blvd., Suite 1101
Los Angeles, Calif. 90010
(213) 382-2353

Togo
Togo Information Service
1706 R St., N.W.
Washington, D.C. 20009
(202) 667-8181

Trinidad & Tobago
Trinidad & Tobago Tourist Board
118-35 Queens Blvd.
Forest Hills, N.Y. 11375
(718) 575-3909

Tunisia
Embassy of Tunisia, Tourist Affairs Section
1515 Massachusetts Ave., N.W.
Washington, D.C. 20005
(202) 862-1850

Turkey
Turkish Consulate General
General Office of the Culture & Information Attaché
821 United Nations Plaza
New York, N.Y. 10017
(212) 687-2194

Uruguay
Uruguay Consulate, Tourist Information
747 Third Ave., 37th Floor
New York, N.Y. 10017
(212) 753-8191

U.S. Virgin Islands
U.S. Virgin Islands Division of Tourism
3450 Wilshire Blvd., Suite 915
Los Angeles, Calif. 90010
(213) 739-0138

Yugoslavia
Yugoslavia National Tourist Office
630 Fifth Ave., Suite 280
New York, N.Y. 10111
(212) 757-2801

Zambia
Zambia Airways, Tourist Information
400 Madison Ave.
New York, N.Y. 10022
(212) 685-1112

A Tourism Miscellany

The following is a list of guidebooks and other information sources related to disabled travel.

Accent Special Publications
Box 700
Bloomington, Ill. 61702
 ["Going Places in Your Own Vehicle" booklet]

Access Travel
Consumer Information Center
Pueblo, Colo. 81009
(800) 948-3334

Accessibility Information Center
National Center for a Barrier-Free Environment
Suite 1006
1140 Connecticut Ave., N.W.
Washington, D.C. 20036
 [A list of guidebooks for handicapped travellers]

Canadian Rehabilitation Council for the Disabled
Suite 2110, One Yonge St.
Toronto, Ontario, Canada M5E 1E5
 [*Handi-Travel: A Resource Book for Disabled and Elderly Travellers*]

Evergreen Travel
Betty Hoffman
4114 198th St. SW
Lynnwood, Wash. 98036
(800) 435-2288 or (206) 776-1184

Information Center for Individuals with Disabilities
Fort Point Place, 1st Floor
27–43 Wormwood St.
Boston, Mass. 02217
(617) 727-5540
   [Offers useful problem-solving assistance, including travel agents who specialize in tours for the disabled]

Itinerary
P.O. Box 1084
Bayonne, N.J. 07002
(201) 858-3400
   [Bimonthly travel magazine for the disabled]

Langlois Medical Escort Services
P.O. Box 51418
Durham, N.C. 27717
(800) 628-2828
   [Traveling nurses]

LTD Travel
116 Harbor Seal Court
San Mateo, Calif. 94404

Mobility International
P.O. Box 3551
Eugene, Ore. 97403
(503) 343-1284
   [Membership organization with annual fee]

Northern Cartographic Dept. AA
P.O. Box 133
Burlington, Vt. 05402
(802) 655-4321
   [Access America special atlas for disabled; also national park guides]

Palex Tours
P.O. Box 33015
Haifa 31033, Israel

Rehabilitation International U.S.A.
1123 Broadway, Suite 704
New York, N.Y. 10010
(212) 620-4040
[International Directory of Access Guides, a compendium of
publications on accessibility to cities, transportation systems,
and hotel chains]

Society for the Advancement of Travel for the Handicapped
26 Court St., Suite 1110
Brooklyn, N.Y. 11242
(718) 858-5483

Travel Information Center
Moss Rehabilitation Hospital
12th Street and Tabor Road
Philadelphia, Pa. 19141
(215) 329-5715

Travel Industry Disabled Exchange (TIDE)
5435 Donna Ave.
Tarzana, Calif. 91356
(818) 343-6339

Twin Peaks Press
Box 129
Vancouver, Wash. 98666
(206) 694-2462
[Publishes several useful resources, including *Travel for the
Disabled*, *Directory of Travel Agencies for the Disabled*, and
Wheelchair Vagabond]

Wes Johnson
Wide World Travel
1640 Camino del Rio North
San Diego, Calif. 92108

Athletics and Recreation

The following organizations and associations offer support for athletic and recreational endeavors of a wide variety of types. These organizations are frequently headquartered in members' homes rather than regular offices. Because of that, some organizations may not list phone numbers and prefer written inquiries.

4-H and Youth Development Extension Service
Room 3860-S
U.S. Department of Agriculture
Washington, D.C. 20250
(202) 447-5853

52 Association
Bori Rauchmann
441 Lexington Ave., Suite 502
New York, N.Y. 10017
(212) 986-5281
  [Ski program for amputees]

Access to Recreation
2509 E. Thousand Oaks Blvd., Suite 430
Thousand Oaks, Calif. 91360
(800) 634-4351 or (805) 498-7535 (in Calif.)
  [Catalog of adaptive recreation equipment]

American Alliance for Health, Physical Education and Recreation
  for the Handicapped
Information and Research Utilization Center
1201 16th Street, N.W.
Washington, D.C. 20014

American Alliance for Health, Physical Education, Recreation and
  Dance
1900 Association Drive
Reston, Va. 22091
(703) 476-3400

American Athletic Association of the Deaf
3916 Lantern Drive
Silver Spring, Md. 20902

American Blind Bowling Association
150 N. Bellaire Ave.
Louisville, Ky. 40206

American Blind Bowling Association
c/o Gilbert Baqui
3500 Terry Drive
Norfolk, Va. 23518
(804) 857-7267

American Camping Association
5000 State Road
Martinsville, Ind. 46151
(317) 342-8456

American Wheelchair Bowling Association
Robert Moran, Exec. Sec.
6718 Pinehurst Drive
Evansville, Ind. 47711
(812) 867-6503

American Wheelchair Pilots Association
Dave Graham
P.O. Box 1181
Mesa, Ariz. 85201

Amputee Sports Association
George Beckmann, Jr.
P.O. Box 60129
Savannah, Ga. 31420-0129
(912) 927-2756

A/V Health Services, Inc.
Cindy Collet Hodges
P.O. Box 20271
Roanoke, Va. 24018
(703) 772-0659 or (703) 389-5724
  [*Wheelchair Aerobics* video]

Boy Scouts of America, Scouting for the Handicapped
1325 Walnut Hill Lane
Irving, Tex. 75038-3096
(214) 659-2127

California Wheelchair Aviators
Fritz Krauth, Pres.
12570 Brookhurst St., #5
Garden Grove, Calif. 92640
or
117 Rising Hill Way
Escondido, Calif. 92025
(619) 746-5018

Canadian Recreational Canoeing Association
P.O. Box 500
Hyde Park, Ontario
Canada N0M 1ZZ0

Canadian Wheelchair Sports Association
333 River Road
Ottawa, Ontario
Canada K1L 8B9
(613) 748-5685

Committee for the Promotion of Camping for the Handicapped
830 Third Ave.
New York, N.Y. 10022
(212) 940-7500

Disabled Boater and Camper News
R.D. Miller
H.B.D.S. News Co.
P.O. Box 73
Lyons, Ill. 60534
(708) 839-0505
  [Newsletter covers Midwest and comes out six times a year]

Disabled Sportsmen of America
P.O. Box 5496
Roanoke, Va. 24012

Disabled Outdoors
5223 South Lorel Ave.
Chicago, Ill. 60638
(312) 284-2206
  [Quarterly newspaper]

Handicapped Scuba Association
1104 El Prado
San Clemente, Calif. 92672
(714) 498-6128

Indoor Sports Club
1145 Highland St.
Napoleon, Ohio 43545
(419) 592-5756

International Braille Chess Association
c/o H. H. Cohn
128 Walm Lane, Willesden Green
London NW2 4RT
England

International Committee of the Silent Sports
Gallaudet College
800 Florida Avenue, N.E.
Washington D.C. 20002
(212) 651-5144

*International Directory of Recreation Oriented Assistive Device
Sources*
Lifeboat Press
P.O. Box 11782
Marina del Rey, Calif. 90292
(213) 305-7474
  [Emphasis on mobility impairment]

International Foundation for Wheelchair Tennis
Peter Burwash
1909 Ala Wai Blvd, Suite 1507
Honolulu, Hawaii 96815
(808) 946-1236

International Foundation for Wheelchair Tennis
2203 Timberloch Place, Suite 126
The Woodlands, Texas 77380
(713) 363-4707

International Games for the Deaf
Langaavej 41
DK-2650 Hvidovre, Denmark

International Sports Organization for the Disabled
Stoke Mandeville Sports Stadium
Harvey Road
Aylesbury, Buckinghamshire
England

International Wheelchair Road Racers Club
16578 Ave., N.E.
St. Petersburg, Fla. 33702

Let's Play to Grow
1350 New York Ave., N.W.
Suite 500
Washington, D.C. 20005-4709
(202) 393-1250

Michigan Amputee Foundation
Terry Willis
6849 So. Division Ave.
Grand Rapids, Mich. 49508
  [Low-impact aerobics video]

N.S.S.R.A.
636 Ridge Road
Highland Park, Ill. 60035
(312) 831-2450

National Amputee Golf Association
24 Lakeview Terrace
Watchung, N.J. 07060

National Amputee Athletic Association
Dick Bryant, President
836 Oakwood Terrace
Antioch, Tenn. 37013

National Association for Sports for Cerebral Palsy
66 E. 34th St.
New York, N.Y. 10016
(212) 481-6359

National Archery Association
1750 E. Boulder St.
Colorado Springs, Colo. 80909
(719) 578-4576

National Foundation of Wheelchair Tennis
Brad Parks, Dir.
3857 Birch St., Suite 411
Newport Beach, Calif. 92260
(714) 669-1453

National Handicapped Sports
1145 19th St., N.W., Suite 717
Washington, D.C. 20036
  [*Fitness Is for Everyone* video]

National Handicapped Sports and Recreation Association
Capitol Hill Station
P.O. Box 18664
Denver, Colo. 80218
(303) 632-0698

National Junior Horticultural Association
c/o American Horticultural Society
P.O. Box 0105
Mount Vernon, Va. 22121
(703) 768-5700

National Park Service
Division of Special Programs and Populations
Department of Interior
18th & C Street, N.W.
Washington, D.C. 20240
(202) 343-4747

National Therapeutic Recreation Society
3101 Park Center Drive
Alexandria, Va. 22302
(703) 820-4940

National Wheelchair Athletic Association
3617 Betty Drive, Suite S
Colorado Springs, Colo. 80917-5993
(719) 574-1150

National Wheelchair Basketball Association
110 Seaton Bldg.
University of Kentucky
Lexington, Ky. 40506
(606) 258-8784 or (606) 257-1623

National Wheelchair Marathon
Paul DePace
380 Diamond Hill Rd.
Warwick, R.I. 02886
(401) 738-7304

National Wheelchair Softball Association
Dave Van Buskirk, Commissioner
P.O. Box 737
Sioux Falls, S.D. 57101

National Wheelchair Racquetball Association
c/o AARAA
815 Weber, Suite 203
Colorado Springs, Colo. 80903

National Wheelchair Roadracer's Association
Jackson Memorial Hospital
1611 N.W. 12th Ave.
Miami, Fla. 33136

New York City chapter
National Multiple Sclerosis Society
30 West 26 St., 9th Floor
New York, N.Y. 10010
  [*M.S. Workout* video]

North American Riding for the Handicapped Association
Leonard Warner, Exec. Dir.
Box 100
Ashburn, Va. 22011
(703) 777-3540 or (703) 471-1621

Paralyzed Veterans of America
801 18th Street, N.W.
Washington, D.C. 20006
(202) 872-1300

Reach Foundation
Orthopedic Hospital
P.O. Box 60132
Los Angeles, Calif. 90060
(213) 742-1332

Recreational Mobility, Inc.
P.O. Box 147
Elmira, Ore. 97347
(503) 935-2828

Janet Reed
12275 Greenleaf Ave.
Potomac, Md. 20854
  [*Wheelchair Workout* video]

Resources for Artists with Disabilities, Inc.
60 East Eighth St., Number 289
New York, N.Y. 10003
(212) 460-8510
  [Established by DAA member Lois Kaggen of New York City]

Royal Bee Corporation
703 Kihekah
Pawhuska, Okla. 64056
(918) 287-1044
  [Electric fishing reel]

Ski For Light
c/o Bud Keith
737 North Buchanan St.
Arlington, Va. 22203
(202) 245-6671

Slabo Productions
1057 So. Crescent Heights Blvd.
Los Angeles, Calif. 90035
[*Keep Fit While You Sit* video]

S'PLORE (Special Populations Learning Outdoor Recreation and
Education)
699 E. South Temple, Suite 120
Salt Lake City, Utah 84102
(801) 363-7130

Special Olympics
1350 New York Ave., N.W.
Washington, D.C. 20006
(202) 628-3630

Sequoya Challenge
P.O. Box 1026
Nevada City, Calif. 95959

Project SNAP (Special Needs Adapted Photography)
Polaroid Corp.
784 Memorial Dr.
Cambridge, Mass. 02139
(617) 577-2000

Stuart's Sport Specialties
7081 Chad St.
Anchorage, Alaska 99502
(907) 349-8377

U.S. Amputee Association
Richard Bryant
Route 2, County Line
Fairview, Tenn. 37062
(615) 670-5453

United States Deaf Skiers Association
Two Sunset Hill Road
Simsbury, Conn. 06070
(203) 658-7456

United States Quad Rugby Association
311 Northwestern Drive
Grand Forks, N.D. 58201
(701) 772-1961

Vinland National Center
P.O. Box 308
Loretto, Minn. 55357
(612) 479-3555 (Voice or TTY)
  [Gives physical education/sports courses, publishes guides about
  sports and physical fitness; videotapes can be rented for small
  fee.]

Wheelchair Motorcycle Association
101 Torrey St.
Brockton, Mass. 02401
(617) 583-8614

Windy City Disabled Outdoors Club
2102 W. Ogden Ave.
Chicago, Ill. 60612
Contact Nick Coletta, (312) 744-7229, or Judy Benson, (312)
  525-8636

World Recreation Association of the Deaf
P.O. Box 7894
Van Nuys, Calif. 91409

Miscellaneous Resources

Use of One Hand, or Other Limited Hand Use

Handbook for One-Handers
Federation of the Handicapped
211 West 14th St.
New York, N.Y. 10011

Single-Handed: A Book for Persons with the Use of Only One Hand
Accent Special Publications
P.O. Box 700
Bloomington, Ill. 61702

The Typing with One Hand Manual
Fred Sammons
P.O. Box 32
Brookfield, Ill. 60513
(312) 325-1700

Firms that Adapt Vehicles for Mobility Impaired Persons

Once again, the list presented here is not intended to be exhaustive; rather, it is presented to give you suggestions of places to begin looking for assistance in your part of the country.

Braun Corporation
Phone (800) 843-5438 for dealer nearest you

Howard Burkett
The Rincon Corp.
11684 Tuxford St.
Sun Valley, Calif. 91352

Cameron Enns Company
P.O. Box 5019
Fresno, Calif. 93755
(209) 222-2922

Drive-Master
16A Andrews Dr.
West Paterson, N.J. 07424
(201) 785-2204

Freewheel Vans, Inc.
4901 Ward Rd.
Wheat Ridge, Colo. 80033
(303) 467-9981

Gresham Driving Aids, Inc.
P.O. Box 405
Wixom, Mich. 48096
(800) 521-8930

Handicapped Driving Aids of Michigan, Inc.
4020 Second St.
Wayne, Mich. 48184
(313) 595-4400

Handicaps, Inc.
4335 So. Santa Fe Drive
Englewood, Colo. 80110
(303) 781-2062

Kroepke Kontrols
104 Hawkins St.
Bronx, N.Y. 10464
(212) 885-1100

Haveco
421 Amity Rd.
Harrisburg, Pa. 17111
(800) 692-7293 (Pennsylvania only) or (717) 238-1530

Mednet, Inc.
544-546 WaWeeNork Dr.
Battle Creek, Mich. 49016-0948
(616) 962-3800

Mobility Products and Design, Inc.
3200 Harbor Lane
Minneapolis, Minn. 55441

New Era Transportation, Inc.
810 Moe Drive
Akron, Ohio 44310
(216) 633-1118 or (800) NET-VANS
  [Vans, driving adaptions, lifts, extended tops and doors, parts,
  service and repairs on all models]

Smithermans, Inc./Orthopedic Appliance Co., Inc.
Birmingham, Ala.
(205) 324-2579 or (205) 322-0384

Tri-State Mobility Equipment Co.
940 Cleveland Ave. S.W.
Canton, Ohio 44707
(216) 489-6666

Vartanian Industries, Inc.
P.O. Box 636
Switzgable Dr.
Brodheadsville, Pa. 18322
(717) 992-5700 or (212) 863-7043

Wells-Engberg Co.
P.O. Box 6388
Rockford, Ill. 61125
(800) 642-3628

W.R. Davis Engineering Ltd.
1260 Old Innes Road
Ottawa, Ontario, Canada K1B 3V3
(613) 748-5500
    [Quick-release hand controls for automobiles.]

A book on this subject, *Going Places in Your Own Vehicle*, is available from Accent Special Publications (P.O. Box 700, Bloomington, Ill. 61702). Also, check with the nearest Center for Independent Living for assistance/suggestions.

Home Modification

"Adaptable Housing"
United States Department of Housing and Urban Development
P.O. Box 280
Germantown, Md. 20874-0280

American Institute of Architects
1735 New York Ave., N.W.
Washington, D.C. 20006
(202) 626-7475
    [Free bibliographies of material on barrier-free design]

American National Standards Institute
1430 Broadway
New York, N.Y. 10018
(212) 642-4990
  [Ask for Pamphlet No. A117.1 1986]

Architectural and Transportation Barriers Compliance Board
1111 18th St., N.W.
Washington, D.C. 20036
(202) 653-7834
  [Independent federal regulatory agency charged with ensuring
  the accessibility of certain facilities]

Association of Physical Plant Administrators
1446 Duke St.
Alexandria, Va. 22314
(703) 684-1446
  [Books on large-building modification]

Barrier Free Environments
P.O. Box 30634
Raleigh, N.C. 27622
(919) 782-7823
  [A design company]

Eastern Paralyzed Veterans Association
432 Park Ave. South
New York, N.Y. 10016
(212) 686-6770
  [Free "Wheelchair House Designs" booklet]

Housing and Home Services for the Disabled
Home Design by Maxine Atwater
500 23rd St. N.W., Suite 308
Washington, D.C. 20037

How They Grow: A Handbook for Parents of Young Children with Autism
The National Society for Children and Adults with Autism
1234 Massachusetts Ave., N.W., Suite 201
Washington, D.C. 20005
  [Sources of information and services for modifying a home
  (N.Y. area)]

J & S Kogen Builders, Inc.
Joel Kogen, Vice President
P.O. Box 1700
1755 Lake Cook Road
Highland Park, Ill. 60035
(708) 831-0066 or 831-3300
FAX: (708) 831-3337
  [Specialists in building for disabled and senior citizens]

National Task Force on Life Safety and the Handicapped
c/o Edwina Juillet
1015 15th St., N.W., Suite 700
Washington, D.C. 20005
(202) 347-5710

New York State Office of Vocational Rehabilitation
(800) 222-5627
  [Designs, builds, and finances home modifications for disabled workers]

United Cerebral Palsy, Project Open House
1770 Stillwell Ave.
Bronx, N.Y. 10469
(212) 519-5181
  [Free home modifications; some restrictions apply]

Index

Pharos Books are available at special discounts on bulk purchases for sales promotions, premiums, fundraising or educational use. For details, contact the Special Sales Department, Pharos Books, 200 Park Avenue, New York, N.Y. 10166.